Praise for *Stop Pain*

*"If there is one thing I hate, it is physical pain of any kind. That is why I value Dr. Vad and his book **Stop Pain** so much. His advice on eating, exercise, alternative treatments, and medical options are truly helpful. I am not only a patient of Dr. Vad, I'm a fan."*

— **Joy Behar,** comedian and host of *The View*

*"Vijay Vad is about as kind, caring, and smart a physician as is possible to find in this modern age. He wants all of us to suffer less pain. And, with this book, he gives readers the same good advice he offers in his sports medicine practice at New York's famed Hospital for Special Surgery. **Stop Pain** is empowering, wise, and helpful. It's the next best thing to seeing this fine doctor yourself."*

— **Claudia Dreifus**, science journalist and author of *Interview* and *Scientific Conversations*

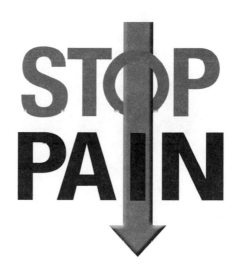

Also by Vijay Vad, M.D.

Arthritis Rx: A Cutting-Edge Program for a Pain-Free Life

*Back Rx: A 15-Minute-a-Day Yoga- & Pilates-Based
Program to End Low Back Pain*

*Golf Rx: A 15-Minute-a-Day Core Program
for More Yards and Less Pain*

Published and distributed in the United States by: Hay House, Inc.:
www.hayhouse.com • *Published and distributed in Australia by:* Hay House
Australia Pty. Ltd.: www.hayhouse.com.au • *Published and distributed in the
United Kingdom by:* Hay House UK, Ltd.: www.hayhouse.co.uk • *Published
and distributed in the Republic of South Africa by:* Hay House SA (Pty), Ltd.:
www.hayhouse.co.za • *Distributed in Canada by:* Raincoast: www.raincoast.com •
Published in India by: Hay House Publishers India: www.hayhouse.co.in

Design: Jami Goddess
Interior photos: William G. Cahill: **williamgcahill@gmail.com**
Interior illustrations: Eric Angeloch: **angeloch@earthlink.net**
Indexer: Jay Kreider

Library of Congress Cataloging-in-Publication Data

Vad, Vijay.
  Stop pain : inflammation relief for an active life / Vijay Vad, with Peter
Occhiogrosso.
     p. cm.
  Includes bibliographical references and index.
  ISBN 978-1-4019-2525-3 (hardcover : alk. paper) 1. Pain. 2. Pain--Treatment. 3.
Exercise therapy. 4. Self-care, Health. I. Occhiogrosso, Peter. II. Title.
  RB127.V33 2010
  616'.0472--dc22
                                     2010000271

ISBN: 978-1-4019-2525-3

13 12 11 10   4 3 2 1
1st edition, May 2010

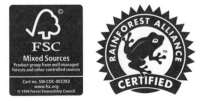

Printed in the United States of America

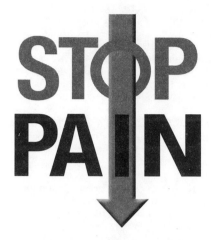

STOP PAIN

Inflammation Relief for an Active Life

VIJAY VAD, M.D.

with Peter Occhiogrosso

HAY
HOUSE

HAY HOUSE, INC.
Carlsbad, California • New York City
London • Sydney • Johannesburg
Vancouver • Hong Kong • New Delhi

I dedicate this book to my son, Nikhil, who managed to smile through pain from a very young age. May he and his sister, Amoli, be inspired to continue the work of the Vad Foundation for a more peaceful and prosperous world.

Contents

Introduction

Some days when I was in the thick of creating this book, I would schedule a little time at the end of my workday to write and edit my manuscript. But the end of the day never seemed to come. Patient after patient was added to my schedule until I barely had time to get home to my family and eat dinner. A lot of the patients I see are suffering from some kind of chronic pain condition, and even as the number of new technologies and medications to treat pain grows year by year, the number of people in pain seems to grow even faster. Each year, an estimated 50 million Americans suffer from chronic pain—any condition that persists for more than six months—and an additional 25 million suffer from acute pain. Two-thirds of these 75 million patients have been living in pain for more than five years, and treating their conditions has cost a quarter of a trillion dollars during those five years. According to the American Pain Foundation, persistent pain is the second leading cause of medically related work absenteeism, resulting in more than 50 million lost workdays each year.[1]

About one-third of all chronic sufferers describe their pain as being almost the worst pain they can possibly imagine. And their pain is more likely to be constant than flaring up frequently. Only about half of people with chronic pain say their pain is nearly under control, and that applies primarily to those with moderate pain. The majority of those with the most severe pain do not have it under control, and among those who do, it took almost half of them over a year to reach that point. We really shouldn't be surprised, then, to learn that the most commonly prescribed medication *of any category* in the United States is hydrocodone, a powerful, potentially addictive painkiller.[2]

We don't have to look very far for the causes of this explosion in chronic pain, not only in the U.S. but worldwide as well. Obesity plays a bigger role in creating pain than most people realize; more than one-third of adults in the U.S.—over 72 million people—and 16 percent of U.S. children are obese. Since 1980, obesity rates for adults have doubled, and rates for children have tripled. Now, for the first time since these statistics have been kept, the percentage of Americans rated obese is *higher* than those merely considered overweight; the combined rate is a staggering 65 percent.[3] Despite everything we have learned about the dangers of fast food and processed food, refined sugar and trans fats, the numbers of overweight and obese people continue to rise globally. Along with increasing your risk for heart disease, adult-onset diabetes, and cancer, being overweight or obese puts increased stress on all the lower body joints, including the hips and knees as well as the lumbar spine, or lower back. And all that leads to ever more cases of chronic pain.

The major cause of this epidemic of obesity, along with our increasingly sedentary lives, is the standard American diet (with the apt acronym SAD). The double-whammy here is that the elements of the SAD also tend to promote inflammation, relying as they do on high-calorie, sugar-and-salt-laden food and snacks; fast and processed food, with a preponderance of sweeteners and additives derived from corn; and other inflammatory vegetable oils and syrups. As we'll see in great detail in this book, inflammation is one of the leading causes of chronic pain—although that connection is only now beginning to be recognized by medical researchers.

Along with poor diet and resulting obesity, another deadly duo is adding to our pain: excessive stress and inadequate deep sleep. Stress—created by a high-paced lifestyle, increasing economic burdens, and a wide range of environmental toxins from noise to air pollution—is itself a factor in creating pain. Although some psychological or physical stress is needed for proper body function, too much stress is bad. Excessive psychological stress causes the body to secrete a powerful but potentially destructive hormone called cortisol, which is associated with the "fight or flight" response. The body is designed to handle the occasional stress response to danger, but prolonged levels of cortisol in the bloodstream impair cognitive ability, thyroid function, and immune response. Cortisol can also cause blood sugar imbalances, decrease bone density and muscle mass, raise blood pressure, and increase abdominal fat, which is associated with heart disease and stroke.

As if all that weren't bad enough, chronic stress robs us of sufficient deep, restorative sleep. The inability to unwind and escape from stress tends to interrupt what sleep we get, never allowing us to sleep deeply for long enough. The profoundly restful period of deep REM (rapid eye movement) sleep, the time when we dream most actively, is also the time our bodies need to repair and renew themselves.[4]

For all these reasons, and despite the array of expensive, hi-tech machinery and costly prescription medications, a higher percentage of the population is suffering from chronic pain now than ever before. We could probably say that drugs like hydrocodone aren't part of the solution but part of the problem.

The Hospital for Special Surgery (HSS) is one of the premier venues in the country for the treatment of musculoskeletal ailments and injuries, with a long list of star athletes among its patients. As a sports medicine specialist at HSS for the past 15 years, I have seen my share of professional and college athletes, but many of my patients are ordinary citizens suffering from the same kind of chronic pain that probably drove you to pick up this book: arthritic knees and hips, painful spinal injuries, frozen shoulder, tennis elbow, and various other degenerative musculoskeletal conditions.

One thing I've learned in my many years of treating chronic pain is that a low-tech, traditional, minimally invasive approach can often get better results than invasive surgery. Even back in medical school I sensed that we relied too much on technology and the orthodoxy of Western medicine, and not enough on establishing a relationship with each patient and following our instincts as healers. We were taught to be precise and do everything by the book, and that has its place. But the best doctors I've known are healers first.

My ideas about medicine and healing were shaped to some extent by the culture in which I came of age. I grew up in a large city in the western part of India called Poona (now known as Pune), a city much like Boston, with many small, top-notch colleges. But despite the availability of sophisticated conventional medical care, many people relied on the ancient science of Ayurvedic medicine for any number of ailments. Ayurveda, a system of traditional medicine native to India, stretches back several thousand years, yet remains influential throughout much of South Asia today. The ailments for which people have sought Ayurvedic remedies were not necessarily life-threatening illnesses like heart disease or cancer, but everyday problems and health issues, from an arthritic joint to simple nausea. The value and potency of some of these remedies were clear to me even as a young child. When I was two or three years old, my maternal grandfather had lymphoma, and he was treated at Tata Memorial Center, named for a great Indian philanthropist, in Mumbai (Bombay), which is the Indian equivalent of Memorial Sloan-Kettering Cancer Center in New York. There my grandfather underwent lengthy courses of chemotherapy and radiation that eventually healed his cancer, but the treatments had such debilitating side effects, including significant pain, that he looked worn and was essentially bedridden, unable to do anything. Granddad was an avid gardener who enjoyed spending four to six hours in the garden every day; now he couldn't even get out of bed, which was distressing to him.

So my grandfather decided to seek out an Ayurvedic doctor, who prescribed an herbal preparation. This wasn't some cheap folk concoction; the doctor had to travel many miles to locate the proper herbs, which then had to be heated in water at a specific temperature for a precise amount of time at home. I can still remember the smell, which was god-awful. Yet after a few weeks of drinking this Ayurvedic tonic daily, not only did my grandfather recover from the effects of chemo and radiation, but his vigor and health also returned fully. His lymphoma went into remission, and he was fine for the next 15 years. He felt that the Ayurvedic preparation helped heal his cancer and keep it in remission for all those years. Though we'll never truly know what role it played in his cancer, the remedy clearly made a difference in helping him cope with the chemo and radiation. Even in conventional medicine, many drugs have their origins in herbs or roots, like aspirin, which is essentially a willow bark extract. And in the last decade, leading medical institutions, such as Johns Hopkins, have begun investigating the potential therapeutic effect of various herbs on different cancers.

Perhaps because I was so young when I saw my grandfather find relief in Ayurveda, I feel more open to it than other doctors. The fact that an Ayurvedic preparation had helped my grandfather feel much better when the hospital treatments were making him so sick imparted a lasting impression on me. My parents, both of whom are physicians, appreciated the use of natural remedies as well. They would give us ginger and clove for sore throats and nausea. Ginger is a miracle drug that doesn't get a lot of attention from pharmaceutical companies, because you can't patent it. Nonetheless, it has been used for centuries in India with great success—and it has no side effects. My paternal grandfather suffered from arthritis brought on by a hockey injury. But he used yoga and incorporated ginger into his daily diet to counteract pain and inflammation, and maintain a mobile life until a ripe old age.

Even though I came from a family of doctors, I didn't get serious about medicine until we moved to the United States, specifically to Norman, Oklahoma, and I became an undergraduate at the University of Oklahoma in 1984. Not long after I entered medical school there, I started to see the shortcomings of the medical system in this country. I realized, for instance, that we spend a lot of money researching exotic technologies, based largely on the profit motive—expensive machines and high-end drugs can earn billions of dollars a year for technology and pharmaceutical companies. And because of these incentives, the medical world often bypasses some of the most tactical, low-tech solutions that can still have a big impact. A prime example is exercise therapy, or physical therapy, which can be extremely effective in healing musculoskeletal injuries. I still believe that walking a minimum of

30 minutes daily is one of the best health maintenance activities you can do.

Some physicians do recommend physical therapy for their patients who are experiencing chronic pain, but they are just as likely to suggest surgery or prescribe high-risk medications. While these conventional remedies can help, they often make the problem worse. And although I was trained to rely on these treatments, over time I began to trust more in my instincts and what worked best for my patients, including exercise regimens based on yoga and Pilates, along with recommendations for proper diet and nutritional supplements.

Dietary supplements derived from natural herbs and plants, like the ginger that helped my grandfather overcome the pain from his arthritic knee, have amazing medicinal value. There is nothing exotic about these remedies, many of which have been tested in clinical studies around the world. As we'll see in a later chapter, medications derived from natural sources can have as great a healing impact as medicines that take pharmaceutical companies years to develop and may cost hundreds of dollars for a month's supply. They also often have far fewer associated risks.

Ultimately, I began researching my own set of safe, low-tech alternatives to the prescription and over-the-counter (OTC) pain medications currently on the market. In the process, I formed a research consortium called the Inflasoothe Group (inflasoothe.com), in conjunction with my friend Richard LaMotta, an inventor, entrepreneur, and philanthropist. Over a period of five years, we developed a topical cream and oil designed to be available without a prescription, called The MD System oil and cream. The clinical trials performed on these topicals using a group of amateur golfers revealed that 64 percent of participants had significant pain relief compared to placebo, and 70 percent reported improved golf performance and less back pain. My research group now includes scientists with doctorates in the areas of pharmacy, materials science, and rehabilitation. We are also researching a new generation of creams, oils, skin patches, drinks, and exercise machines that are designed to curtail inflammation while restoring mobility. Because in the end, relieving pain comes down to learning how to reduce the factors that increase your body's sensitivity to pain, such as a pro-inflammatory diet, lack of exercise, and dependence on prescription medications. At the same time, you have to multiply the factors that decrease pain sensitivity, such as an anti-inflammatory diet, deep breathing, aerobic exercise, and healing supplements without side effects.

But first, you'll need to know something of the complex mechanism behind pain so that you'll understand why certain conventional treatments offer little relief, while other, often simpler treatments are more successful. We know so much more about what causes pain than we did just 10 or 20 years ago, and that new knowledge can help you alleviate pain without doing damage to other parts of your body.

For that reason, we'll begin in Part I with an explanation of the ways in which your body experiences various kinds of pain and which factors tend to increase or decrease your sensitivity to it. We'll also look at what I consider to be the most important, yet largely ignored, truth about pain: its link to inflammation. And I'll explain why it's so important to locate the precise cause of your pain, so you can avoid being labeled with one of the many commonly overdiagnosed syndromes.

Throughout Part II, the heart of this book (and in the related appendices), I'll show you all the things you can do to alleviate pain on your own, even if you are working with a physician at the same time. These essential self-care options include:

- An anti-inflammatory diet that will help reduce your sensitivity to pain.

- Sensible exercise that you can do even when you're suffering from chronic pain.

- Ergonomically sound working and living recommendations that will help you avoid some of the major causes of chronic pain.

- Effective dietary supplements to relieve chronic pain. The drug companies won't tell you about these, and most doctors haven't fully researched them, but these supplements have been used, in most cases, for hundreds of years with no significant side effects!

- Common OTC medications, including pills, patches, and topical creams and gels. You'll learn the good and the bad—how they work and the possible dangerous side effects.

- Techniques to help you cope with the 12 most common pain problems.

I'll lay out the most promising options for integrative care in Part III, explaining safe, complementary pain treatments, such as physical therapy, massage, osteopathy, chiropractic, and acupuncture. We will also look at the all-important mind-body connection, and how you can use the power of meditation, visualization, deep breathing, and talk therapy to counteract chronic pain and the feelings of depression or hopelessness that often accompany it.

Then in Part IV I'll tell you what you need to know about the relevant conventional medical options that are offered by many doctors to chronic pain sufferers. If you are currently taking or thinking of taking prescription pain medications, you should at least know all the potential dangers and drawbacks before you do. The same goes for a list of medical procedures, including various surgeries. We've been programmed to value surgical intervention, and indeed, in many life-threatening situations from heart disease to cancer, surgery can seem like a godsend. But when it comes to relieving chronic pain, many elective surgeries may not be necessary, and can possibly do more harm than good. I'll describe the basics of several common procedures and surgeries, and outline the alternatives.

Finally, in Part V, I'll answer a few of the most frequently asked questions I field from my patients every day. This part of the book amounts to everything you ever wanted to know about pain but were afraid to ask. No question is too small or too trivial. (For instance, is there truth to the popular saying "No pain, no gain"?)

A FEW WORDS (MOSTLY UNDER THREE SYLLABLES) ABOUT MEDICAL LANGUAGE

In medical school they say that you learn the equivalent of six foreign languages in the first two years. Maybe that's stretching it a bit, but medical jargon is so unfamiliar and interdependent that when you're introduced to one new medical term you have to learn ten other new words to understand what the first one means. In that sense it *is* a foreign language, even though it's English. But because I know how it feels to get acclimated to a new language, I don't want to subject you to that awkward sense of floating in a strange world, like being underwater without a scuba tank and face mask. For that reason, I've tried to simplify the medical language and put almost everything into layman's terms, but without oversimplifying. When a medical term is useful and has no lay counterpart, I'll stop to explain it before moving on. You should be able to understand what I'm talking about without having a medical dictionary nearby. The important thing is that you're able to grasp what I'm saying so that you can apply it directly to your own life and healing your pain. That's always my primary objective.

PART I

PAIN

Chapter One

What Is Pain?

Early one Sunday morning, I was just finishing breakfast when my emergency pager went off. It was a recent patient of mine, whom I'll call John. I had been working with John for several months on alleviating a chronic pain condition that he'd had for more than seven years. We had been able to minimize his pain levels with a regimen of proper diet, exercise, supplements, topical creams, and minimally invasive procedures. This morning, however, he was experiencing an especially disturbing "breakthrough pain," a condition that affects many chronic pain sufferers. Breakthrough pain comes on suddenly for short periods of time and can't be alleviated by the patient's normal pain management arsenal.

I have seen breakthrough pain due to bumps in the road of everyday life—factors that alter the mind-body relationship. Common culprits are extreme stress, or excessive flying, as the pressurized cabin in the plane can take a toll, or something as simple as catching a cold, which can trigger breakthrough pain by increasing overall inflammation in the body. It is common in cancer patients, but it also happens occasionally for the kinds of people I treat—those suffering mainly from musculoskeletal pain, or MSK for short. Many researchers and physicians now prefer to use the term *neuromusculoskeletal pain*, because it accurately suggests that the nervous system is not only involved but also fundamentally altered by such pain, sometimes irreversibly. I'll follow their usage (although for simplicity I'll retain the traditional acronym MSK), because to understand how pain works, we have to assess the role played by the exceedingly complex human nervous system.

Indeed, most of the pain people suffer from, both in this country and in other parts of the world, involves the complex system of nerves (*neuro*), muscles and tendons (*musculo*), and bones, joints, and cartilage (*skeletal*). MSK pain, which covers a wide range of symptoms and causes, affects one in four adults worldwide and is the most common source of serious, long-term pain and physical disability. Chronic pain, often a result of unresolved MSK pain, is the cause for as many as 60 percent of people requiring early retirement or long-term sick leave. The costs associated with treating this form of pain in the United States alone reached a quarter of a trillion dollars during the years from 2003 to 2008. Excluding trauma, MSK conditions are responsible for roughly 25 percent of the total expense of illness in all developed nations. The monumental impact of MSK conditions is now recognized by the United Nations, the World Health Organization, the World Bank, and numerous governments throughout the world that support the Bone and Joint Decade 2000 to 2010. According to an influential paper released in 2008, this form of pain is "one of the most common reasons for self-medication and entry into the health-care system."[1]

My patient John may be just one small part of those statistics, but to me he represents the personal side of pain, because I saw just how big of a toll it took on his daily life. When I met John, he was at his wit's end, having all but given up hope of getting relief from what he experienced as "round the clock" pain. John runs several successful computer programming and Internet technology companies that require him to drive fairly long distances to work. When he first came to see me several years ago, the long drives were causing him considerable back pain. John is now in his mid-40s, but the initial source of his pain was an injury that occurred when he was just 14. While competing in a karate tournament, he threw a roundhouse kick, also called a "720" because it requires two full

4

revolutions of the leg and body to deliver the blow. His opponent had fallen against the ropes to get out of the way, however, so there was nothing to stop John's leg and lower body from continuing to spin out of control. The whiplash left him a little sore, but he was able to finish the match. He didn't feel bad that day, but the pain soon intensified.

"I woke up the second day after the tournament," John said, "and I was absolutely screaming for my mother." At the hospital, he was given traction and sent home the following day. John felt essentially normal for the next ten years, with only an occasional backache. He spent a decade laying tile and granite floors for a living, and even though he was on his knees most of the day, John felt little back pain, because his work forced him to maintain a strong body core and tight stomach. The problems developed after he stopped doing manual work and started his first computer job. He had been going to night school while laying tile, but once he began working at a computer station full time, he lost his core body tone, and after a few years his back pain started in earnest.

After examining John, I determined that he had a tear in the soft tissue in one of his spinal discs. When healthy, the discs separating the vertebrae in your spine are like jelly donuts: they have soft, gel-like centers surrounded by layers of fibrous tissues. Because of injury or aging, small tears can form in the outer layer of the disc (this is called an "annular tear"). When the gel-like center of the disc pushes through—like squeezing the jelly out of the donut—the result is a herniated disc. John had sustained a tear on the outside lining of a lumbar disc, located in the lower back. This caused inflammation of the nerve going down his left leg and resulted in severe back and leg pain.

The tear was most likely the result of that missed karate kick, and had gradually worsened over the years. John had seen a doctor in Florida who gave him an annual selective nerve root block (SNRB) injection, which is a special form of epidural injection commonly used for diagnosis and back pain management. The SNRB injections worked for a year or so, and John occasionally saw a chiropractor. But as his life became more sedentary and he put on more weight, the frequency of the injections went from once a year to every nine months, then six months, then three, and finally every two weeks. John was on what you might call a pain roller coaster.

CHRONIC VS. ACUTE PAIN

In a strange way, we in the West have developed a kind of split personality about pain. We may not like feeling it much, but we sometimes are taught that we should "suck it up" and bear it. I don't believe that's helpful, and in fact, just the opposite may be true. Some research has shown that pain and suffering can be extremely deleterious to our health, and not simply by making it hard for us to concentrate on work or family, or by reducing the quality of our lives. John C. Liebeskind, a renowned pain expert and a professor of psychology at UCLA, found that pain can even kill by delaying healing and causing cancer to spread.[2]

Part of the misunderstanding about pain may come from the confusion between acute pain and chronic pain. Acute pain—say, from a severe burn or deep cut—may cause intense suffering, yet the pain is temporary. Just knowing that it will pass makes such pain more bearable. The pain incurred by a broken limb may be excruciating, but we can take solace in the day-by-day mending process and the gradual lessening of hurt and discomfort. Once the cast comes off, we usually feel relieved and whole again. In this case, complaining about the pain may indeed be counterproductive; we should do what we can to relieve the pain but focus primarily on healing its cause.

Chronic pain is often less intense than acute pain, but nonetheless can be far more debilitating. Thinking that there seems to be no end to this kind of pain makes it more difficult to bear on a psychological level. In this situation, it may be necessary to attack the painful symptoms as much as their cause. For one thing, the longer we suffer from a particular form of chronic pain, the lower our pain threshold becomes. This means that it takes less stimulation to initiate a feeling of intense pain. Just think of a bruised knee that you keep reinjuring. Merely pulling on a pair of pants can become a painful act, because the pain threshold has become so low. For that reason, we must be careful to treat acute pain quickly and effectively, so that it doesn't evolve into chronic pain. If the tear in his disc had been correctly identified and treated earlier, John would have saved himself a lot of suffering.

In this book, I will be talking about both acute and chronic pain, although I'll be spending more time on chronic pain for a number of reasons. After all, you can use many of the same treatments to reduce acute pain that I will be describing for chronic pain. And most acute pain can be treated effectively by conventional and/or integrative modalities that are commonly available, including physical therapy, acupuncture, and chiropractic. Cuts, burns, stings, breaks, and sprains are considered "self-limiting," which means that as the painful stimulus lessens—you take your hand off the object that is too hot or cold, or your leg is placed in a cast and neutralized—the pain decreases markedly. Often even a severe pain in the low back or along the sciatic nerve in the leg will disappear as inexplicably as it occurred. (Some such pain may actually be cyclical, meaning that it will come and go.) Chronic pain, meanwhile, is both more complicated and more mysterious. It generally develops through a cumulative series of smaller changes we make to cope with acute neuromusculoskeletal pain. The chronic MSK conditions that most commonly require treatment include arthritis, back pain, and tendonitis. The incidence of chronic MSK pain is expected to increase substantially as levels of obesity continue to grow, not only in the developed world but in emerging nations as well. As our society ages and the baby boom generation enters their 60s, we can expect to see an exponential explosion in chronic MSK pain, so it really pays to know how it's caused and what we can do to stop it.

Chronic pain, which, as noted earlier, is defined as lasting more than six months, is most often caused by a failure to effectively treat some form of acute pain. Many of us have suffered acute pain at some point in our lives, whether from a bruised muscle, sprained ankle, broken bone, deep cut, or serious burn. But as long as the acute pain from those injuries is diagnosed and treated quickly and properly, we are generally able to avoid having it develop into chronic pain. Early intervention is the key—but not too early. Many conditions will heal themselves in six to eight weeks with modified activity and common sense treatments, such as ice, heat, soothing balms, and OTC medications. (See Appendix A for information on treating acute pain.) But after that time, if the injury hasn't healed and the pain dissipated, what are known as "pain pathways" are formed and lead to chronic pain.

Chronic pain can also be the result of an ongoing condition, such as arthritis, defined as the loss of cartilage—the shock absorbers in the joint—that can produce painful inflammation in the joints and limit range of motion. In other cases, it may be caused by an illness, such as a chronic Lyme disease infection, or even surgery that damages a nerve.

Chronic MSK pain, as with other chronic pain conditions, may be the result of a past injury, but it can also be due to the buildup of everyday stresses. A slipped or bulging disc as described above, for instance, may be the result of being overweight. But there may be other stresses on the disc, such as extended sitting, as with writers, artists, and office or factory workers, or driving. Truck drivers further compound the risk factor of driving long distances with lifting during loading and unloading.

Genetics and age also play prominent roles in chronic MSK pain. As we age, the gel within our spinal discs tends to dry out, making the spine less flexible and more prone to traumatic injury. And the relative strength of the protective outer layer of our discs is also conditioned to some extent by our genetic history in much the same way as some people are predisposed to cancer or diabetes. Being overweight can also increase the risk of our discs drying out.

And yet, chronic pain can sometimes be mysterious, its root cause hard to determine. There may be no evidence of disease or damage to tissues that doctors can directly link to pain. Or pain may remain after the original injury shows every indication of being healed—as was the case with John's karate injury and resulting acute back pain. John saw seven different doctors, including back and pain management specialists, orthopedic surgeons, osteopaths, and chiropractors, yet any relief he felt was always short term. "Nobody really seemed to spend any time to talk with me," he said.

"It was like a mill. You were in there for fifteen minutes and then you were out. You got a prescription and you were gone—and that drove me insane."

The prescriptions he got were for NSAIDs (non-steroidal anti-inflammatory drugs); nerve membrane stabilizers originally designed for seizure control; painkillers including opioids; and muscle relaxers. He was even given a complicated procedure called a nucleoplasty, which in his case wasn't called for. The problem was that the main source of his pain was the tear in the disc and not the bulge itself, which nucleoplasty is designed to treat. One specialist he saw even talked about replacing the damaged discs altogether.

When John finally came to see me, he was not only in pain but also feeling a great deal of frustration verging on despair. He told me that he was experiencing pain from the time he woke up in the morning until he went to sleep at night, and that the pain often disturbed his sleep as well. Even with all the treatments and medications he had gotten, he just wasn't getting significant relief. He could not sit for even five minutes—a hallmark clinical sign of a tear in the disc.

I decided to approach his situation from all directions. The weight he had put on and the prolonged sitting he endured during his years of sedentary work had added enormously to the initial problem of his injury. So I started John on a weight loss regimen of aerobic exercises, including swimming, treadmill walking, and yoga-based stretching exercises (See Appendix B for a selection of these stretching exercises) and an anti-inflammatory diet. I also advised him to make other lifestyle changes, such as cutting down on his commute and heating his back for 15 minutes at bedtime and in the morning and icing it after work. I told John that if he did all these things, he would see a significant improvement within six months. In a very short time, John went from missing two or three days of work per week because of his pain to being able to work five days a week.

To help him with the pain he felt while driving or flying long distances, I recommended a back brace designed to take pressure off the low back. The combination of using the brace for prolonged sitting, 45 minutes of daily walking and the weight-loss regimen was helping John start to break the pain cycle. I also gave him samples of an OTC patch and topical cream that managed to further reduce his pain during his daily commute and while at work.

It's not that John has no pain at all now. We are managing his pain in an ongoing way and keeping it at a minimum. I may still occasionally prescribe anti-inflammatories or pain meds, or suggest going to an osteopath, but only when absolutely necessary and only for short periods. I am usually able to get many patients to a pain-free stage pretty quickly, but others who have been seriously injured or have gone untreated for lengthy periods of time have to be willing to stay in it for the long haul. John knows that if he maintains the regimen he'll do all right most of the time. And that's a big change from the way he felt when all he experienced was pain. As he once put it, "When I'm in so much pain, I feel like I'm in the middle of a crowded room screaming and no one hears me. When you're in round-the-clock chronic pain, you feel lonely and isolated."

Knowing that there is a way out of pain and that people care about you is a major source of comfort at times like that. My job as a physician was not to treat him and his various scans as numbers in a generic protocol, but to customize his treatment plan, because pain is personal.

THE PATHWAYS OF PAIN

Over the years, writers and researchers have used many different metaphors to try to describe how pain works and how pain messages travel from the point of injury to the brain. One of the original theories of pain, the specificity theory, stated that there was a direct line of communication that ran from the skin or inner organs to the brain, and that the intensity of the pain would be directly related to the intensity of the injury to the affected tissue or organ. The origins of the specificity theory can be traced back at least as far as 1664 when the French philosopher René Descartes likened how pain messages travel to a man pulling on a rope attached to a bell. Just as the bell rings with a pull from afar, the brain reacts to a specific distant stimulus that sends information along a specific pain pathway.[3] The specificity theory was modified somewhat during the 19th century by the understanding that different sensations (touch, warmth, cold, pain) are conveyed by different nerves, even different kinds of nerves, and that the quality of sensation is determined by how and where these nerves interact with the brain. But by the beginning of the 20th century, this traditional theory of pain was so fully accepted in medical school systems that it was actually being taught as fact instead of theory.

During this same time, though, evidence started accumulating that the theory of a "direct-line communication system" did not adequately explain how we perceive pain. For one thing, surgically severing any of the nerves along the pain pathway did not stop patients from feeling pain. Then, in 1959, the Harvard anesthesiologist Henry K. Beecher wrote about seriously wounded soldiers who reported much lower levels of pain, even when they had suffered severe tissue damage in combat, than his civilian patients in the recovery room of Massachusetts General Hospital. Some of these soldiers, Dr. Beecher reported, had "entirely denied pain," despite the obvious evidence of their injuries. The men may have exhibited one form of pain control through positive thinking, because injury meant that the soldiers would be allowed to go home or at least be taken out of combat and so sustain no further injury. Or they may have been distracted by other, more powerful concerns, such as staying alive or protecting their comrades. In any event, the notion of a direct correlation between a noxious or harmful stimulus and an accompanying sensation of pain was clearly off the mark.[4]

That was our first solid hint that there was much more to pain than any simplistic theory could explain. Later researchers produced what is known as the gate control theory, which said that a "gating" mechanism within the back part of the spinal cord (called the dorsal horn) opened up when nerve fibers that carry pain sensations transmitted a high volume and intensity of pain, but closed in response to normal stimulation of the nerve fibers that transmit sensations of touch that we recognize as relief. This would explain why, among other things, rubbing the site of an injury provides some immediate comfort.

The gate control theory also opened other possibilities for controlling pain of all sorts. The "gates" that controlled the brain's perception of pain could be closed in a variety of ways, from pain-killing drugs and injections to mind-generated techniques such as meditation, visualization, and biofeedback, with many other modalities in between. Something as simple as taking a 30-minute walk while listening to your favorite music can help initiate endorphin release and control pain as effectively as more complicated procedures or medications in many cases. (I'll have more to say about the role of endorphins in Chapter Five.)

HOW YOU FEEL PAIN

Imagine that you are sautéing some vegetables in olive oil in the kitchen, using a stainless steel skillet. Just as you turn off the burner, the telephone rings. You go into the living room to retrieve your phone, and then come back in the kitchen. Distracted by the call, you grab the skillet with your other hand. That's when you suddenly feel a searing pain. Instinctively, you let go of the frying pan, which falls back onto the stovetop, but not before spilling some of the hot oil onto your leg. Putting down the phone, you rush to the sink to run cold water over your hand, but by now the oil is also starting to scald your leg. Grabbing some paper towels, you wipe the hot oil from part of your leg, and continue rubbing even after it's gone, because the sensation feels comforting and is relieving some of the more intense pain caused by the scalding oil. After telling your friend you'll have to call back, you assess the damage. The hand that picked up the hot skillet hardly hurts at all, somewhat numbed by the cold water. Your leg, meanwhile, hurts quite a bit. You go to the freezer to get some ice cubes to put in a plastic bag and apply this improvised ice pack to your throbbing leg. As several blisters appear on your leg, you wonder whether you need to call your doctor.

So what exactly happened during your accident? What caused you to feel pain? Why did your body respond differently to two related events? What can you expect to feel as time goes on?

We can simplify this complex process by identifying the major components of the nervous system that play a role in causing and relaying the sensation of pain. Think of this as a system of pain pathways that acts as a two-lane highway, with traffic moving simultaneously in both directions, often at extremely high speed. The initial pain signal goes up one side of the highway, through the spinal cord, and arrives at the brain, which functions like a kind of dispatch office. The pain signal then returns down the other side of the highway. Anywhere along that two-lane highway, we have the ability to increase or decrease sensitivity to pain.

But the painful journey begins with special pain receptors— nociceptors—that are sensitive to harmful stimuli. They do not react to non-painful stimuli; these nociceptors are stimulated specifically by actual or threatened injury to tissue. If not for their sensitivity, you might hold on to the hot skillet until your skin begins to blister and you sustain serious, possibly permanent damage. Pain receptors are most concentrated in areas that are prone to injury, such as fingers and toes, but they are prevalent throughout your entire body. They are also connected to muscles and internal organs, for instance, where they serve the same function of starting the message of pain on its journey to your brain.

After the nociceptors sense a stimulus, they send a message to your peripheral nerves, which extend from the skin, muscles, and internal organs to the spinal cord. These nerves are made up of individual nerve cells, or neurons, that, when stimulated, relay a chemical (called a neurotransmitter) or electrical signal from one to the next in extremely short bursts of time—somewhere between three and nine one-thousandths of a second—which makes possible our rapid reaction to intense pain.

Nerves attach to the spinal cord, itself a soft bundle of nerves that runs from the base of the brain to the lower back, at the dorsal horn, which runs along the back of the spinal cord. After the alert about the hot skillet handle travels from the pain receptors to the

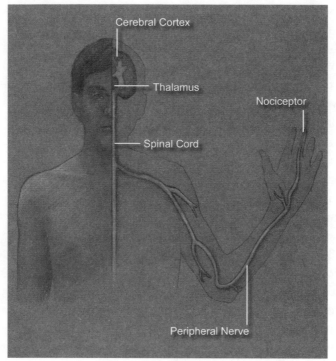

Fig. 1. The Nerves

dorsal horn of the spinal cord, it is passed along to the thalamus, an area of your brain responsible for processing and relaying sensory information selectively to other parts of the brain. The thalamus determines which signals to dispatch to the cerebral cortex, which is like the traffic control center where we make our decisions and manage the movements of our limbs, sometimes involuntarily. It forwards the pain message simultaneously to three areas of the brain:

- The somatosensory cortex, which records and responds to physical sensations

- The limbic system, which generates emotions

- The frontal cortex, which creates thoughts and thought patterns

Working in concert, these areas of the brain respond by sending messages that increase or decrease the level of pain in the spinal cord in different ways. Some signals travel on to the motor cortex, then back through the spinal cord to the nerves and down the highway to the point where the pain occurred. These impulses cause the necessary muscle movements to respond to the source of pain—in this case, letting go of the hot skillet. Other signals are sent back along descending highways that have neurons that can "intercept" additional ascending nerve signals both in the brain and spinal cord, so these don't register as pain. In other words, they can cut off the pain messages before they are recognized as pain, like police setting up a roadblock! This produces pain relief, or *analgesia*. Your brain may also signal nerve cells to release natural pain relievers known as endorphins—which also cause that euphoric feeling many people get from doing aerobic exercise—and help diminish the pain messages.

In some cases, unfortunately, nerves may release chemicals that *intensify* the pain, a process called *sensitization*, which lowers your pain threshold and can result in chronic pain. During sensitization, your nervous system amplifies and distorts pain for reasons that aren't entirely clear. Sensitization can also result from inflammation, which causes your pain receptors to fire with greater intensity, for a longer time, and at a lower threshold.

Sensitization may affect all the pain-processing regions of your nervous system, including the sensing, feeling, and thinking centers of your brain. When this occurs, chronic pain may be associated with emotional and psychological suffering. Because pain and emotional sensation share the same pathways, moreover, chronic pain sensitization can cause changes in brain chemistry that not only magnify the severity of the pain but also may lead to clinical depression.[5]

Researchers know, based on observation, that the brain somehow influences pain perception. For example, the searing pain you felt in your hand quickly lowered in intensity once you let go of the handle, and subsided further as you held it under the cooling water. But if you could take your mind off the pain in some other way (deep breathing, visualization, biofeedback), it would bother you even less. This implies a link between pain and cognition, and we'll take a closer look at this in Chapter Eleven on the mind-body connection.

We already know from numerous scientific studies that patients given placebos (dummy pills) for pain control often report that the pain diminishes or stops altogether, even though the pill has absolutely no analgesic, or pain-relieving, content. This kind of evidence indicates that somewhere along the highway, between the point where the pain originates and the dispatch center in the cortex where the message arrives through your nerves, or on its return trip to the part of your body that initiated the pain message, your perception of pain can be changed. In some cases it may be made worse, and in others alleviated.

Pain researchers are now focused on identifying the biology that underlies sensitization, as well as other genetic and psychological factors that determine how you feel pain. Inflammation at the site of injury may add further to your pain, and is one area that is receiving special scrutiny. In the next chapter, we'll examine this relationship between inflammation and pain in greater detail.

Chapter Two

The Link Between Inflammation and Pain

Colleen suffered from mild low-back pain. We had been treating her successfully with a combination of stretching exercises, supplements, and dietary modifications. But then she caught a virus and the pain in her back shot way up. I prescribed a dose of ibuprofen twice a day for two weeks, which helped reduce the acute flare-up of pain she had been experiencing. Colleen couldn't understand why the viral infection affected her back pain. After all, the two problems are totally unrelated, aren't they? Though this seems to be the case, there was a link between them—*inflammation*. The viral infection caused an inflammatory response throughout her entire body, which added to the low-level inflammation of her back pain and sent her over her pain threshold. I couldn't blame Colleen for her confusion—physicians themselves are only now becoming aware of the link between inflammation and pain, and many still don't fully grasp its implications.

Understanding the role that inflammation plays in causing and intensifying pain is perhaps the most radically important development in pain treatment that has occurred in the last decade or so. Researchers have known for some time that despite all the life-saving benefits of inflammation—the body's reaction that aims to remove foreign invaders and start healing—this protective process comes with potentially debilitating side effects. In a delicate kind of dance, the body's immune system must turn on the inflammatory response—heat, swelling, redness, pain—as soon as possible after experiencing a harmful infection or injury, but then turn it off once the process has accomplished what it was designed to do. Unfortunately, this doesn't always happen, and our graceful dance partner can suddenly become a treacherous adversary.

To complicate matters, inflammation often develops insidiously over time in response to a combination of factors, including wear and tear on your joints and spine or toxic elements in your environment and diet. Any linkage of short-term and long-term causes for inflammation—say, a knee injury accompanied by a flu infection and a pro-inflammatory diet—increases the risk of developing chronic pain. It's essential to know how your immune system generates and oversees your inflammatory response, so that when it doesn't turn off at the appropriate time, you can take action. The more familiar you are with the rhythms and stages of your body's inflammatory reaction, the better chance you have of making it work for instead of against you. You also need to learn how to work with it, as you would with any dance partner: if you make the right moves and avoid certain missteps, you will experience much less pain.

THE COMPOUNDING TRIGGERS OF INFLAMMATION

Inflammation has many causes, and their effects are cumulative. Some triggers may be local (a bruised knee or shoulder, a bulging disc), but others may be systemic manifestations, like a flu virus or a sudden increase in mental stress. For example, many studies have established a correlation between MSK pain and depression. It's not always clear which problem came first, the pain or the depression, but there is no doubt that mental stress and depression can be inextricably intertwined with chronic pain. The pain from a herniated disc may also become more severe when compounded with other physical problems in the spine, or situational factors, such as poor posture or prolonged sitting. As the various causes of inflammation build up, they develop a kind of negative synergy. It's a little like having people constantly asking you for money: You can handle a few reasonable requests from relatives, business associates, or even strangers on the street. But when everyone you know demands money from you every day, and then your property taxes go up and your adjustable mortgage payments keep increasing, your standard of living is going to decrease, and eventually you may even go bankrupt.

Let's say you already have incipient arthritis in your low back or knee caused by a gradual wearing away of the cartilage, as happens to many of us over time. But then you have to take several plane trips on business, and the changes in pressure from ascending and descending in the plane's pressurized cabin trigger an inflammatory response in the joints in your back. Add to that your exposure to an influenza bug on your last flight home, and in your weakened condition you come down with a viral infection. Now your entire system undergoes an inflammatory response.

Or, let's say you didn't have to take all those plane trips, but you've been eating the kind of standard American diet that is loaded with pro-inflammatory foods (we'll talk more about those in Chapter Four). That can also cause systemic inflammation as your digestive tract and circulatory system respond to the toxins in all that fast food and processed food. Alternatively, you may live in a city with a polluted environment, breathe recycled air in your office and automobile fumes on the streets; or maybe you live in the countryside near high-tension wires or a coal-fired power plant. In these cases the toxins in the air evoke an inflammatory response from your respiratory system. Finally, all those years of lifting heavy objects at the factory, unloading your truck, carrying firewood, or even just playing golf and tennis in every spare moment all add stress to your joints. Your immune system might be able to handle any one or two of these risk factors, but when you keep piling them on, both locally and systemically—bad diet, toxic air, viral and bacterial infections, cabin pressure, wear and tear on your cartilage and the discs between your vertebrae—it's too much for your system to handle. It all amounts to what we might call a synergy of pain.

This negative inflammatory synergy may eventually mushroom from a relatively manageable ailment like an arthritic lower back to a systemic malady, such as diabetes, cancer, or heart disease. So the sooner you learn to recognize the presence of inflammation in relationship to your pain, the better chance you will have to decrease, and perhaps terminate, both.

THE INFLAMMATORY CASCADE

As you know, inflammation is part of the immune system's network of protection against foreign invaders, injury, or a cumulative degeneration in the cartilage or spinal discs. The inflammatory response is far from simple, however. It consists of a complex, multilevel reaction in which one event flows naturally from another, like an elaborate series of waterfalls. For that reason, physicians and researchers speak of this self-protective response as the *inflammatory cascade.*

The cascade begins with the body's early response to a triggering injury of some kind. After the initial immune response, the inflammatory cascade continues as the first white blood cells—our body's armed forces—arrive on the scene and recruit more cells to increase the system's response to the pathogen, like advance scouts calling for backup. This growing army of immune cells has some positive effects: it slows bleeding and clears away debris from the destroyed tissue. If the tissues are irrevocably damaged, the inflammation process produces scar tissue that keeps other invaders out.

Unfortunately, you can have too much of a good thing, and, as noted earlier, inflammation has its downside. For example, in autoimmune disorders, the body's defense mechanisms turn against substances and tissues normally present in the body, wrongly destroying normal tissue, which often leads to other diseases. It's like a fire that you build in the woods when you're in danger of freezing to death. Once you get the fire going, you warm your hands and feet again, and the threat to your survival is removed. But if you keep your hands near the flames as they grow higher and higher, eventually you're going to get burned. Then maybe the forest catches fire, too, and you have to run for your life!

One of the more common conditions associated with inflammatory cascades that I treat—not to mention one of the best illustrations of this phenomenon—is the bulging spinal disc. To understand the whole process, however, it will help to have a clear picture of the how the spinal column itself functions. The bones, or vertebrae, of the spinal column run down the back, connecting the skull to the pelvis. The column is divided into the cervical spine (neck), the thoracic spine (the part behind the chest), the lumbar spine (lower back), and the sacral spine (the part connected to the pelvis that doesn't move). The letters and numbers that you may see on a radiology report or hear from your physician refer to specifically numbered vertebrae in each of these regions. For instance, C2 is the second cervical vertebra (singular of *vertebrae*) from the top of that part of the spine; L4-5 indicates the fourth and fifth lumbar, or lower back, vertebrae; L5-S1 refers to the fifth lumbar and first sacral vertebrae, and so forth.

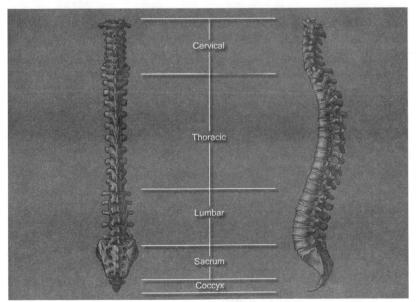

Fig. 2. The Spinal Cord

All of these vertebrae have hollow cores that serve to protect nerves stretching through them from the brain down and out to the rest of the body. The bony vertebrae are separated by flexible discs filled with a soft, gelatinous substance that provides cushioning and balance to the spinal column. In the image of a jelly donut that I used to describe these discs in the last chapter, this substance would be the jelly. Its scientific name is the *nucleus pulposus*, but it doesn't have a common name, so I'll just call it the jelly in the donut. When the harder "skin" of the disc surrounding this jelly (the donut itself, so to speak) is torn in an accident or by continued abrasion, the jelly-like fluid pushes the skin of the disc outward. In extreme cases, the fluid itself leaks out of the tear. This hernia, or rupture, impairs the ability of the disc to cushion the two vertebrae that are above and below it, which is bad enough. But the fluid itself is extremely nerve-hostile. It takes only a small amount of this released fluid to cause tremendous pain to the surrounding nerves by triggering the inflammatory cascade.

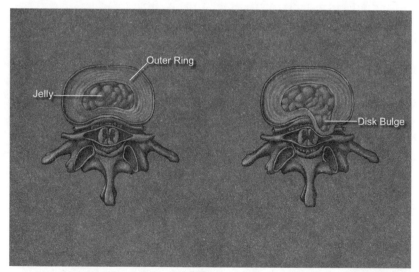

Fig. 3. Normal Disc and Bulging Disc

When the jelly from one of your discs leaks into the spine, it's a little like spilling sulfuric acid on your hand. If that jelly comes close to the nerve, it causes a high level of inflammation that leads to severe pain in your low back. Much more of the pain from a herniated disc comes from this release of nuclear fluid and the resulting irritation of the nerve than from mechanical pressure of the disc rubbing against a nerve.

This is just what happened to Sean, a 28-year-old who was on his honeymoon in Thailand. Although Sean had never done yoga, he took a strenuous yoga class with his wife, and the next day he started to experience severe pain in his left leg. By the time Sean landed back in New York, the leg pain was so intense that he could hardly sit. He came to my office directly from the airport. We got an MRI that showed an L5-S1 left-sided disc bulge—meaning the jelly from the donut between those two vertebrae had leaked toward his left side, causing severe nerve inflammation. Considering his acute level of pain and disability, I gave Sean an epidural injection of triamcenelone (a corticosteroid with 50 times the anti-inflammatory potency of ibuprofen). Within three days his pain was 90 percent diminished. The pain was caused not by pressure from the bulging disc, but by the inflammation resulting from release of the disc jelly, which the corticosteroid neutralized.

In Sean's situation, many doctors would recommend surgery as the surest way to relieve pain and restore full range of motion. The medical rationale for most back surgery to relieve spinal pain is that a herniated, or bulging, disc is creating "pressure" on a nerve, the spinal cord, or a nerve root. But the latest research is beginning to show that back pain and related leg pain are only partly caused by compression, more so by chemical inflammation, as in the case with Sean. Research has also focused on tears in the outer coating of the spinal disc—the ring of the donut I referred to above, called the annulus—which contains many nerve fibers. These annular tears can lead to chronic pain and substantial loss of quality of life.

LEVELS OF INFLAMMATION

The level of inflammation in your body has a direct influence on the level of pain. In general, the lower the inflammation, the less pain you experience. Let me give you some examples of circumstances in which increasing inflammation can have a direct impact on pain.

The response of our immune system is at its highest level in cases of infection, whether from a virus, such as the flu, or from an infected wound; the inflammation level is not quite as high in autoimmune diseases, such as rheumatoid arthritis; and it is only moderately high in chronic conditions including MSK pain, cancer, diabetes, and heart disease. When you come down with the flu or a staph infection, for instance, your inflammation level is on red alert—and you can feel it in every part of your body. As you are attacked by dangerous pathogens including viruses and bacteria, your immune system triggers an extremely potent inflammatory response with which it fights off and kills the foreign invaders. This is the most perilous and immediate scenario confronting the immune system, and it typically responds with all the resources at its command. You may run a fever as the inflammatory response works hard to kill off the invading pathogens. Your muscles and head may ache, and you feel so bad all over that you pretty much want to stay home and stay in bed—which is what you *should* do, so that your immune system can use all its available energy to kill off the invaders. Once the threat is gone, the immune system ideally ceases the inflammatory response, and the level of pain correspondingly diminishes until you feel as good as ever.

The response level in autoimmune diseases, such as rheumatoid arthritis, Crohn's disease, or multiple sclerosis, is not quite as high as in infection, nor is the overall level of pain. We could say that the inflammation level is on yellow alert in this scenario, but the problem is that it tends to stay that way: with autoimmune ailments, an overactive immune system initiates a high inflammatory response that turns against substances and tissues normally present in the body. In essence, the body attacks its own cells under the mistaken impression that they are invaders—a form of "friendly fire" on a massive internal scale. These ailments may be restricted to certain organs—for example, Graves' disease attacks the thyroid—or involve entire bodily systems, as in rheumatoid arthritis or MS. Autoimmune diseases are generally treated through immunosuppression, medication that decreases the very high immune-mediated inflammatory response. With these kinds of diseases, you may be able to function to some extent, but you will still experience a degree of pain much of the time.

When it comes to MSK pain, along with other ailments including heart disease and cancer, the immune system triggers moderate inflammation in a somewhat more limited role to help heal an injury, and then turns it off once it's no longer needed. But when, for a variety of complicated reasons, inflammation runs amok, especially in situations involving chronic pain, it begins to undermine the body in ways that prolong and intensify the sensation of pain. With these conditions, such as osteoarthritis of the knee, hip, or shoulder, or disc problems in the spine, inflammation does not actually turn against the body and begin to attack it as it does with an autoimmune disease. But it lingers and not only causes physical pain but also can affect you emotionally and psychologically, often leading to clinical depression. These debilitating aspects of excessive chronic inflammatory response are what most concern me in finding ways to diminish or eradicate chronic pain. (Although certain autoimmune diseases, such as rheumatoid arthritis, can also give you chronic knee and back pain, those ailments require much more complicated levels of treatment and are not the focus of this book.)

Chapter Three

Finding the Source of Pain

Growing up in India and the United States, I played competitive tennis, and I loved the game with a passion. But during my teen years I suffered a stress fracture in my leg. A stress fracture usually involves a very small crack in the bone, which is why it's sometimes called a "hairline fracture." This kind of fracture typically occurs in weight-bearing bones, such as the tibia in the lower leg, or the bones of the foot, and they often cannot be detected on X-rays. At first, I wasn't sure where my pain was coming from, because unlike with a broken arm or leg, you don't feel a clean break. All I knew is that the pain was so debilitating that I couldn't even walk a block without doubling over. Fortunately, I was diagnosed quickly with a bone scan, and within 12 weeks I was back playing tennis.

For the first four weeks I was on crutches, and the lack of mobility combined with the intense pain when I tried to put any weight on the leg made a huge impression on me. It was the first time I had felt almost helpless and in need of high-grade medical assistance. Through the doctors who treated me, I was exposed to the field of sports medicine, which is devoted to eliminating pain and restoring mobility. And as a direct outgrowth of that whole experience, I became extremely interested in sports medicine as a potential career choice. Because both of my parents are physicians,

I had had significant exposure to medicine while growing up. But this experience brought home to me in a visceral, personal way how valuable sports medicine could be. The pain was personal in the sense that I not only couldn't play a sport I enjoyed, but could not even walk a few feet without excruciating pain. The other thing that the experience impressed on me was the importance of getting the right diagnosis as quickly as possible. I was fortunate that the doctors who treated me at the University of Oklahoma College of Medicine's department of Sports Medicine were very capable, compassionate and caring. And they knew just what they were doing.

THE IMPORTANCE OF A GOOD EXAM

Part of the difficulty of deciding how to treat the pain resulting from a wide variety of MSK ailments is that the precise cause and origin of the pain aren't always immediately clear. I can't emphasize enough how essential it is to understand this, because it can profoundly affect your medical treatment. Unfortunately, the current level of medical evaluation is dictated in large part by medical insurance companies and the most common vehicle for providing health care, the health maintenance organization, or HMO. Many physicians are paid according to how many patients they see within a given time frame, and they may have time for only a brief medical history and cursory exam. As a result, your medical condition may be labeled incorrectly from the beginning, and your treatment plan may never be adequately adjusted to fit the facts of your case.

Still, how well you are diagnosed doesn't necessarily depend on how much money you have or how generous your medical plan is. One of the clearest examples of the importance of taking a detailed history and physical exam involved an extremely wealthy, world-famous philanthropist, whom I'll call Josie, who went to one of the premier medical institutions in the country complaining of pain on the outside of her right knee. The X-rays indicated some early arthritis of the knee, and, based on her complaint, the doctors there took her at her word and injected her knee with cortisone.

The injection, along with prescribed physical therapy, didn't do much to relieve her pain, however, and the next step would have involved arthroscopy for the knee, an invasive procedure. That's when Josie came to see me for a second opinion.

In the course of taking a thorough history, it came out that Josie would limp for a couple of steps whenever she stood up after sitting for a long time. This is an invaluable piece of information, because although that can happen with knee arthritis, it's more indicative of an underlying problem with the hip. To be certain, I gave her not only a thorough knee exam but also a hip exam, and determined that the pain most likely originated from her hip, as hip arthritis often can "refer" pain to the outside of the knee. I ordered radiologic studies of the hip, and they showed early hip arthritis with a degenerative tear in the labrum, a ring of cartilage that surrounds the socket of the hip joint. We injected Josie's hip with cortisone and lidocaine, a local anesthetic. The pain on the outside of the knee disappeared completely—along with the limp upon standing up.

Another thing this story illustrates is that the patient's chief complaint may not accurately identify the source of the pain. Many people can't differentiate between the low back and the hip, for instance, when describing where their pain is located. They may say they have hip pain because they hurt in the area around the hip. But pain from a hip ailment tends to radiate to the front and would be more likely to show up in the groin area. Low back pain radiates into the buttock, but because the sensation of pain may not be centered on the spine, many patients assume it's their hip that's hurting. And in Josie's case, though she could properly identify that the pain was in her knee, the pain she was feeling came from her body adjusting to accommodate MSK pain in a different area. If you properly attend to the hip problem, the knee won't ache from trying to protect the hip. Doctors also have to take into account people's misconceptions or misunderstanding of the root of their own pain.

All of these reasons illustrate why it's so important for the specialist to take a complete medical history and discuss symptoms at length with each patient, and follow with a thorough, hands-on physical exam.

STRUCTURE DOES NOT CORRELATE WITH FUNCTION

Every week I see at least one or two patients whose physician has recommended surgery after examining their radiology. Relying solely on MRIs and X-rays is another major reason that people are often misdiagnosed. While X-rays and MRIs of two patients may look similar, they can be experiencing vastly different amounts of pain. Diagnostic problems arise most often when there is a disconnect between the radiology and the level of pain.

One especially perceptive woman who had had just such an experience liked to say that the doctors she had seen were from the "look at the radiology" school of treatment. That patient, a psychotherapist in her 50s named Barbara, who had a wicked sense of humor, had seen several doctors who were unimpressed after looking at her film (a generic term covering X-rays and MRIs). Barbara had a bulging disc in her lower back, but it looked relatively minor on the MRI. Each of the doctors decided, based on her radiology, that she was not a candidate for surgery. They were being conservative, which is generally preferable when it comes to recommending surgery.

And yet, Barbara knew what she was feeling, and she was in considerable pain. Her back troubles started when she was in her mid-40s. Her son was old enough to go to summer camp, so she suddenly had more free time. "I played tennis all summer and did a lot of gymnastics," she said. "I kept telling myself I felt all right, but two hours later it would really hurt."

After talking to Barbara at length and hearing this story, I realized that she had a classic disc problem. The outward signs of the problem were minimal, just a very small bulging disc, but Barbara was severely debilitated. The pain was not only impinging on her ability to play tennis and golf and go Rollerblading, all of which she loved to do, but it was also making it hard for her to remain seated for more than 15 or 20 minutes. This is a serious problem for someone whose therapy work requires her to sit in a room with clients for upwards of an hour at a time. Barbara was reduced to lying on a couch herself while listening to her patients—a turn of events that might seem funny in a Woody Allen movie but that caused her considerable embarrassment. So when the neurosurgeons who looked at her radiology said that her barely noticeable bulge was too small to operate on, she became enormously frustrated.

After Barbara told me her story, I explained that her experience was proof for a principle you may not find in medical textbooks regarding pain, but that I've discovered to be true after years of working directly with my patients: *Structure does not always correlate with function.* This simply means that the way your musculoskeletal structure looks on your radiology is not necessarily indicative of how it functions and how much pain it actually causes. In her case and others, a relatively small bulging disc can inflict great pain. I recommended that she have a surgical procedure to remove the small bulging disc. She called me two weeks later to say that she was 80 percent pain-free following the procedure.

While Barbara had radiology that didn't indicate the extreme pain she was living with, the structure-function principle also applies in the opposite scenario—when the radiology looks terrible but the pain isn't intense. If fact, this is actually much more common. I would say that about 90 percent of patients who come to me from other doctors have been told that they *should* have surgery, even though less invasive procedures were still available. In many cases surgery is not called for at all, but because the radiology looks bad, that is what the doctors recommend.

Sam, a journalist now in his mid-50s, had a long history of pain in his neck and low back. As a writer, he had lived a fairly sedentary life and had first gone to a chiropractor at the age of 30 because of recurring pain. On the advice of the chiropractor, he began a regular exercise regimen, joining a health club for swimming and weight training; in the winter months he took up cross-country skiing. All those activities should have kept him healthy and strong, but you can also overdo things. Sam liked to split logs for the woodstove in his country home, and that may have exacerbated the effects of an earlier injury. With age, his back and neck pain continued to worsen and he was a regular visitor to the chiropractor, until he began to study qigong (chee-GUNG) in his 40s. An ancient Chinese form of exercise related to tai chi, qigong is less stressful on the back and limbs than yoga, and as a result of following a regimen of low-intensity qigong "forms," Sam was able to stop seeing a chiropractor for the first time in years.

A few years later, however, an X-ray for an unrelated condition revealed severe degenerative disc changes in the cervical (neck) vertebrae and moderate degenerative changes in the lumbar, or low back, region. Concerned, Sam's doctor referred him to a neurologist. After examining Sam, the neurologist ordered a new series of X-rays and MRIs and, based on the results, recommended surgery as soon as possible to repair the damaged discs. Sam thought surgery was extreme and decided to get a second opinion. He saw another neurologist, who examined him carefully and concluded that, although his radiology looked "terrible" and he did have some neck and hip pain, Sam was not incapacitated or experiencing pain radiating to his arms or legs or causing weakness. The neurologist recommended physical therapy with the possibility of a facet joint injection if the PT didn't relieve the pain.

"What about surgery?" Sam asked.

"If I were just looking at your film," the doctor said, "I might be tempted to think so. But my examination shows that there are no neurologic deficits and you have only axial pain." That was his term for low-back and buttock pain, which is a bad prognosis for surgery. "And you still have full use of your arms and legs," he continued. "Because the pain is confined to the areas where the trouble is, we can work with alleviating the pain there. If things get worse in five or ten years, surgery might be an option, but let's not do it now." Ironically, the first neurologist had performed much the same physical examination with similar results; yet he was apparently blinded by the radiology and chose to ignore the fact that his patient still had excellent mobility, no radiating pain, and no neurologic deficits.

Another condition that commonly elicits the prescription of unnecessary surgery is known as "bone on bone," meaning the cartilage in a joint has deteriorated to the point that the bones are making contact without the cushioning effect that cartilage provides. Doctors will say almost reflexively, "Oh you have bone-on-bone arthritis. You need total joint replacement." And yet, I have patients with bone-on-bone conditions who run two or three times a week or play five hours of tennis without pain. Larry is 54 and has a bone-on-bone condition in his knee, yet he could walk long distances without significant pain. He was advised to get a total knee replacement. I told him to take two ibuprofen twice a day only on the days he plays tennis, and he is now able to play several days a week. That's why it's so important not to feel overwhelmed by the results of your radiology report. Just because a doctor or a radiologist's written interpretation of the film says you have bone on bone, a herniated disc, or severe degeneration in one or more spinal discs, that doesn't mean you are condemned to a life of pain or to needless surgery that may actually make your condition worse.

Also remember that pain is subject to change over time, and not always for the worse. Unlike other tissues of the body, our spinal discs receive very little blood supply. Once a disc is injured, it cannot repair itself, and a spiral of degeneration can set in that proceeds through several stages occurring over 10 to 30 years or more. In the early stages, acute pain can make it hard to move normally and have stability. You may experience back pain that varies in intensity, or comes and goes. In the long run, though, your body often *re-stabilizes* the injured segment of the back and you'll experience fewer bouts of back pain that may be less intense when they occur. That's why you should be circumspect before rushing into surgery or other highly invasive procedures.

Because of these kinds of complexities in understanding pain, patients should find a specialist who is thorough and well trained to make a proper diagnosis of the origin of pain. An inaccurate self-diagnosis can conceivably lead to further spinal damage or more severe episodes of MSK pain if the condition is untreated or treated incorrectly. In taking control of your treatment, then, you should continue to work cooperatively with your doctor or doctors. This is the best way to identify the correct location of a disc problem, an ailment in one or more joints, or a strained muscle, and so to determine the full extent of the problem and the actual source of pain.

If I've learned one thing in my years at HSS, it's that pain is very personal. By that I certainly don't mean that pain is only psychological. So, it's vitally important to fit the treatment to the individual patient. That said, of course, only you know best what is working and not working for you, so you have to become involved in your own treatment. I have a patient named Lizzie who injured her knee is a boating accident. Lizzie is a wealthy art collector who travels the world and maintains an active lifestyle in her 60s. One day she was swimming out to meet a Jet Ski to take her to her boat, when a wave lifted the Jet Ski just as she reached it, slamming it into her knee. She eventually lost all the cartilage in that knee and her other as well.

Although Lizzie has been in great pain at times, she loathes the idea of taking painkillers, including most anti-inflammatories and even nutritional supplements. I respect her choices, so we've developed a program that relieves her pain without her needing to take any oral medications. I recommended a regimen of water aerobics, or aquasizing, and breaststroke swimming, which appealed to her because it was active. I give her joint lubricant injections every six months and perform lavage every two years. Lavage (a French word pronounced luh-VAHZH) is a minimally invasive procedure used to wash out any inflammatory fluid or loose debris from inside the joint space. I generally do this using a needle. Then it's an easy matter to remove joint debris using a combination of injected fluid and a small vacuum, rinsing and sucking at the same time. The patient can usually go home one hour after the procedure.

COMMONLY OVERDIAGNOSED PAIN SYNDROMES

The key to a successful diagnosis and treatment is to fit the cure to the specific needs of the patient, being careful to neither overreact nor underreact. That becomes more difficult in the case of pain syndromes that have been inadequately defined or understood by patients and medical personnel alike. A few ailments and their symptoms have been so broadly categorized—in the media, by word of mouth, and even by many physicians—that uncertain doctors and frustrated patients apply them to a dizzying array of pain patterns. Hurried, vague, generalized diagnoses like these are inaccurate a majority of times, which leads to further frustration for patients. Chief among the misdiagnosed or overdiagnosed symptom sets are fibromyalgia syndrome (FMS) and chronic fatigue syndrome (CFS). I see one or two patients every week who have been labeled as having FMS, for instance, based on what I call the "diagnosis of exclusion"—meaning that after the doctors rule out everything else, they say it must be fibromyalgia. Upon a proper history and physical and a review of radiologic studies, I often find that these patients have specific underlying problems that are the cause of their pain, and do not have fibromyalgia at all. Some do, of course, and that makes it all the more important to proceed cautiously. Here are some of the most commonly overdiagnosed syndromes. If your doctor tells you that you have one of these, you may want to go for a second opinion before starting the treatment being prescribed.

Fibromyalgia Syndrome

Patients who come to see me having received a diagnosis of fibromyalgia often turn out to have a specific disc issue in the neck or back, or underlying hip arthritis that's causing the greatest amount of their pain. Yet, because they told their physician that they ache all over, and because the doctor couldn't find any obvious source of their pain, they were diagnosed with FMS. More often than not, I determine that a "pain generator" of some kind is causing their symptoms. By pain generator, I mean the medical "smoking gun," the clearly discernible cause of the pain the patient is reporting. As I said at the beginning of this chapter, that's easier said than done, but through a process of elimination we can usually nail the culprit. Once I locate the pain generator, I can treat that and the symptoms erroneously attributed to fibromyalgia syndrome normally go away. Don't get me wrong: FMS is a real ailment with a specific set of symptoms. It's just that many doctors misdiagnose fibro, because they don't know how to look for pain generators. I'll discuss that process in a moment, but first let me describe what FMS actually consists of.

The term fibromyalgia comes from the Latin word for fibrous tissue (*fibro*) and the Greek terms for muscle (*myo*) and pain (*algos*). Fibromyalgia syndrome is a soft tissue or muscular rheumatism characterized by widespread deep muscle pain, fatigue, depression, and a heightened painful response to gentle touch, focused in multiple "trigger points" or "tender points." Patients may also experience prolonged muscle spasms, weakness in the limbs, nerve pain, a variety of bowel disorders (such as irritable bowel syndrome), and chronic sleep disturbances, during which slow-wave sleep, also called deep sleep, is dramatically reduced. Some skeptics think of fibromyalgia as a manufactured disease, used to fit a loosely defined array of symptoms, or go even further and assume that the patient is a hypochondriac. They blame patients and doctors who can't find an appropriate diagnosis, in part because objective laboratory tests or medical imaging studies are lacking. Still others tend to assign this diagnosis to a broad range of symptoms that are not really related. As so often happens, the truth lies somewhere in between.

I do believe the number of true fibromyalgia cases is much lower than reported. Because women are 10 times more likely to report these symptoms than men, there may also be a subtle bias at work that perceives FMS to be a manifestation of depression or hypochondria. I don't agree with that assumption, but I do concur that both doctors and patients are too willing to apply this name to generalized levels of pain and discomfort. If physicians don't complete a thorough patient history and physical exam, they can easily make a wrong diagnosis. Certain post-viral syndromes, for instance, can cause a condition that sounds like FMS. To be correctly diagnosed with fibromyalgia, a patient has to show specific symptoms, the most important of which is the clear presence of pain in at least 11 of 18 tender points in specific locations on the body. These tender points are located mainly around the base of the neck and shoulders, on the upper outer buttocks, below the elbows, and above the knees. In essence, they are localized areas of tenderness around joints, but not the joints themselves, and they hurt when pressed with a finger. Not deep areas of pain, they are superficial regions that seem to lie under the surface of the skin.

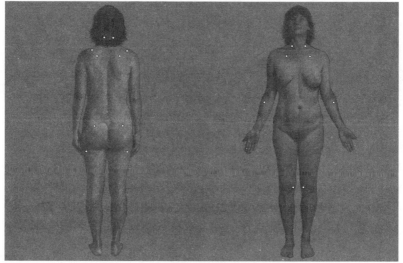

Fig. 4 Fibromyalgia Trigger Points

Once I determine that someone indeed has FMS, I may treat it with neuromembrane stabilizing agents and an antidepressant, but the most valuable treatment regimen is good aerobic exercise. Most of you already know that vigorous exercise can improve your mood, because of the endorphins that are released. What's less well known is that these endorphin releases also powerfully decrease pain sensitivity and lead to higher energy levels. As you might imagine, when people experience pain and hypersensitivity, so that even the touch of a loved one hurts, they become targets for depression. We know that depression and fatigue go hand in hand, so the generalized pain sensations can easily lead to a feeling of not being in control of your life.

Lucille, 47, came to see me having been diagnosed with FMS by a rheumatologist, who had prescribed narcotic painkillers along with both an antidepressant and a neuromembrane stabilizing agent. After a thorough history and physical exam, it was clear to me that most of her pain was in the region of her neck and shoulder blades. She reported that it was worse when she got up in the morning, and she didn't have the other constellation that goes with FMS: the history of depression, irritable bowel syndrome, and 11 of 18 tender points. Apart from being a woman, her biggest risk factor was a relatively stressful job, but pain and stress alone weren't enough to justify the diagnosis.

When I examined Lucille, I found that she had both mild weakness in the nerve root distribution (where nerves pass through the vertebra) with a disc bulge in her lower cervical vertebrae where the neck joins the upper body. She also had what we call "positive spurling," which means that the nerve root and disc bulge were sending shooting pain down into the shoulder blade. When we gave her an epidural injection in her nerve root, her shoulder blade pain went away completely and she had 30 percent relief of her overall pain. Two weeks later we injected the other side and she reported 70 percent overall pain relief. But if you didn't know that this particular cervical nerve root could radiate pain into the shoulder blades, you might have thought she was feeling pain in the tender points located around her shoulders. In addition, some of the fibromyalgia tender points were indeed being hit by the nerve, giving the false impression of FMS when her real problem was a bulging disc.

Chronic Fatigue Syndrome and Epstein-Barr Virus

A number of studies by the Centers for Disease Control and Prevention (CDC) and others have shown that between one million and four million Americans suffer from chronic fatigue syndrome (CFS). Of these at least 25 percent are unemployed or on disability because of their CFS.[1] Astonishingly, only about half of them have ever consulted a physician for treatment, simply assuming that they have chronic fatigue and there is nothing they can do about it. The CDC estimates that about 40 percent of those who report symptoms of CFS have some other previously unrecognized medical or psychiatric condition, such as diabetes, thyroid disease, or even substance abuse. Symptoms of CFS include widespread muscle and joint pain, cognitive difficulties, chronic, often severe mental and physical exhaustion, and other characteristic signs in a previously healthy and active person.

According to one theory, CFS often develops as a *sequela* of the Epstein-Barr virus. (A sequela is any pathological condition resulting from a disease or injury.) The Epstein-Barr virus, or EBV, is a member of the herpes family and one of the most common human viruses. In the United States, upwards of 95 percent of adults between 35 and 40 have been infected, often without serious consequences. Because most people become infected with EBV at some point in their lives, they develop adaptive immunity, preventing repeated sickness from reinfection through EBV antibodies. Yet, EBV is also the pathogen that causes mononucleosis, and may play a role in the neurological degeneration that occurs in people with multiple sclerosis.[2]

Further, a highly publicized 1985 study suggested a strong correlation between EBV and chronic fatigue syndrome.[3] But the CDC points to later studies showing that "many CFS patients have had no exposure to EBV at all."[4]

The best we can say is that although there appears to be a connection between EBV and CFS, not all cases of CFS are necessarily caused by EBV, but may be caused by other viruses or other underlying conditions, such as hormonal problems. EBV can also cause eosinophilia, an increase in certain kinds of white blood cells that is a feature of diseases such as Hodgkin's lymphoma and Gleich's syndrome. In essence, EBV becomes an underlying chronic infection that is hard to cure—a little like having the flu for a year or more. You may not have secondary flu symptoms like nausea, vomiting, or nasal congestion, but you will feel weak and need to rest much more than usual. The worst part is that there is no known cure and you more or less have to let the virus run its course. I knew a 45-year-old psychiatrist who was diagnosed with CFS with very high titers of Epstein-Barr virus in his blood work. (A titer, or titre, is a medical measure of concentration.) As a result, he was so debilitated that he couldn't resume his professional duties for two years.

Chronic fatigue syndrome shares many of the same symptoms as EBV. And, somewhat like FMS, it can be diagnosed by exclusion, but with a different set of parameters. You have to rule out hormonal issues, especially involving the thyroid; underlying depression; and related ailments like Lyme disease, which we'll look at in a moment. Fortunately, the vast majority of patients with CFS will get better over time with proper sleep, aerobic exercise, and proper hydration, even though it may take a few years.

Restless Legs Syndrome

Much like fibromyalgia, restless legs syndrome (RLS) is a currently popular diagnosis that has been overworked and made to account for a wide variety of unconnected symptoms. RLS is a neurological disorder characterized by unpleasant sensations in the legs when at rest and an uncontrollable urge to move in order to relieve these feelings. People have described the sensations as burning, creeping, tugging, or like having insects crawling inside their legs. Ironically, lying down and trying to relax appears to activate the symptoms in most cases, creating a kind of vicious cycle. As a result, most people with RLS have difficulty falling asleep and staying asleep, and the condition can cause exhaustion and daytime fatigue. Again, there is no single diagnostic test for RLS. Although some RLS groups insist that the condition is often misdiagnosed or under-diagnosed, I would say that for every ten patients I see who have been diagnosed with or think they may suffer from restless legs, only one or two actually have the condition. Upon examination, they are more likely to have inflamed nerves in the lower back caused by narrowing of the spaces between vertebrae, damaged nerves, low magnesium levels, or blood circulation deficits. These conditions are important to rule out before making the diagnosis of RLS.

For those with true RLS, I recommend trying a glass of diet tonic water that contains quinine, along with two magnesium tablets around bedtime to be taken for a minimum of eight weeks. Quinine is a mild muscle relaxant that can relieve cramps, and magnesium is a muscle membrane stabilizer that acts synergistically with quinine to minimize symptoms of RLS.

COMMONLY UNDER-DIAGNOSED SYNDROMES

Just as there are a number of commonly overdiagnosed syndromes, others go undiagnosed because doctors are unfamiliar with their symptoms or because the current medical tests are not as sensitive to detection as necessary. However, in the case of both reflex sympathetic dystrophy and Lyme disease, early detection is the key to successful treatment. The longer these syndromes remain undiagnosed and untreated, the more likely they are to lead to chronic pain.

Reflex Sympathetic Dystrophy

Also called complex regional pain syndrome, or CRPS, reflex sympathetic dystrophy (RSD) is a chronic, progressive, and quite painful neurological condition that affects the skin, muscles, joints, and bones. It is essentially a malfunction of part of the nervous system that causes nerves to misfire and send continuous pain signals to the brain. Millions of people in the United States suffer from RSD/CRPS, which affects both men and women, and occasionally children. Although it can occur at any age, it generally strikes between the ages of 40 and 60. The syndrome usually develops in an injured limb in response to an event the body experiences as traumatic, such as a broken arm or leg, or following

41

surgery. However, many cases of RSD result from only a minor injury, such as a sprained ankle, and sometimes no immediate cause is apparent. Patients with RSD/CRPS report dramatic changes in the color and temperature of the skin over the affected limb or body part, accompanied by varying degrees of intense burning pain, pathological changes in bone and skin, excessive sweating, tissue swelling, and sensitivity to touch. Pain may spread unaccountably from one area or limb to another. In some cases, symptoms diminish for a time and then reappear following a new injury.

The Reflex Sympathetic Dystrophy Syndrome Association of America (RSDSA) has determined that the condition develops following one or two percent of bone fractures. Most doctors still aren't certain what causes RSD, however, although genetic predisposition combined with trauma is a strong possibility. One theory suggests that pain receptors in the affected limb become responsive to a family of "fight-or-flight" hormones that are released by the adrenal glands in response to stress. An alternative theory argues that RSD is caused by a triggering of the immune response, which leads to the characteristic inflammatory symptoms of redness, warmth, and swelling.

Early diagnosis of RSD and early intervention are essential to prevent it from causing years of severe chronic pain. This is one of the few pain syndromes for which aggressive early treatment is warranted. Treatments can include medication, physical therapy, psychological support, sympathetic nerve blocks, and spinal cord stimulation. Joseph, a 20-year-old student, sprained his ankle during a pickup football game one Saturday afternoon. By the time he went back to class three days later, his ankle pain had grown worse, and when he saw me, ten days after the injury, his ankle felt warm with significant hypersensitivity. Even when I touched his ankle gently, he screamed as if I were sticking a knife into him. That afternoon, he received his first sympathetic nerve block shot, with a repeat block done a week later. Within four weeks, his RSD had disappeared, and it did not return.

You may be able to detect RSD with a test called a bone scan, which measures metabolic activity. If you catch it right away in such cases, the success rate is high. But time is your enemy, and if RSD is undiagnosed for several months, the success rate goes down accordingly.

I want to emphasize that RSD/CRPS is not a psychological or psychosomatic syndrome. Nevertheless, patients who suffer from it may develop psychological issues when physicians, family, or co-workers do not believe their complaints. The RSDSA reports that because so many health-care professionals are unaware of its signs and symptoms, patients with this disorder see an average of five physicians before being accurately diagnosed. Early diagnosis is important, combined with early intervention. Besides sympathetic nerve blocks, treatment can include the use of nerve membrane stabilizers such as gabapentin or pregabalin; range-of-motion exercises despite pain (RSD is one of the few MSK conditions that requires *working through* pain); and contrast baths—i.e.., heat followed by ice.

Lyme Disease

The bacterium that causes Lyme disease, *Borrelia burgdorferi*, is transmitted among mice, squirrels, and other small animals, and to humans through a variety of ticks. Initial symptoms include headache, fatigue, and a characteristic skin rash. If you don't treat Lyme disease quickly, the infection can spread to joints, the heart, and the nervous system. And in its intermediate and late stages, it can result in arthritis, or nerve damage that may manifest as muscle weakness and loss of balance and coordination, as well as tingling, numbness, cramps, and pain. If Lyme disease is diagnosed properly in its early stage, the usual treatment is a three-week course of antibiotics. But if it goes undetected at first and develops into later stages, a more prolonged course of treatment with antibiotics is usually required, possibly including intravenous antibiotics.

Like the other syndromes I've been discussing here, Lyme disease often eludes diagnosis, and even when you know you have it, the disease can be hard to treat. The transmitting bacterium I mentioned is a spirochete—long, slender, and shaped somewhat like a corkscrew. Although spirochetes are not a large group of bacteria, they can be extremely dangerous, because they are hard to eliminate from your body. They may invade the muscles and joints and the nervous and cardiovascular systems, and they can initiate an anti-inflammatory immune response. Syphilis is also caused by spirochetes, and the two diseases are similar in many ways. Initial symptoms disappear quickly, but if untreated or undertreated, the diseases cause secondary symptoms that become more marked and painful with time. Lyme disease doesn't affect the brain as syphilis does, but it can damage the nerves with increasing severity and cause serious hip arthritis in its late stage. Early diagnosis and aggressive treatment are essential. Sadly, Lyme disease remains under-diagnosed, because current testing is not sensitive enough to detect it.

EARLY DETECTION AND TREATMENT

What I can say unequivocally about all the conditions and syndromes I've discussed in this chapter is that it is crucial to determine their precise origin. Whether we're talking about basic MSK pain caused by arthritis, injuries, or nerve damage, or elusive syndromes that can be hard to nail down, such as fibromyalgia, chronic fatigue, restless legs, or Lyme disease, the key to relieving pain is the same: they have to be diagnosed properly and as early as possible to determine the optimal treatment plan, which should then begin immediately. If you are suffering from one of these conditions and don't feel that the treatments you've been given are relieving your pain, you have to consider the possibility that the diagnosis is at fault and seek a second opinion. Always be willing to question something that doesn't seem to make sense. I'm not talking about self-diagnosis, because that may be a risky business and could cause more harm than good. But if you see a specialist who recommends elective surgery, you need to evaluate all your other options first.

One of the most significant shifts in consciousness regarding health care during the last few decades has been the increasing awareness among the general public, and, to a lesser extent, in the medical profession itself, of the value of patients' involvement in their own treatment. Part of this new understanding involves learning to work with your physician in a proactive rather than passive way. As a patient, you need to know as much as you can about not only your pain but also your treatment options.

Becoming knowledgeable and involved in the process of managing your pain can provide helpful insights that can lead to unexpected results. Another potentially valuable result of taking responsibility for your treatment is the positive sense of empowerment you receive from not allowing yourself to feel like a helpless victim. Just as we have learned from the placebo effect that the mere expectation of healing can produce beneficial results, we should also appreciate the potential healing effect of feeling actively involved in the process.

In the meantime, if you are feeling chronic pain and are in the process of determining its cause, you can do many things to take charge of your healing and pain relief, and, more important, reduce the chances of suffering chronic pain in the future. Whether or not you are under the active care of a doctor at present, there are certain basic courses of action that you can take on your own. Even if you are seeing one or more physicians, all of the information contained in the following chapters will be of value to you. The concept of holistic health doesn't have to be limited to remedies available only in health food stores or over the Internet. Holism means treating your health as a whole, encompassing your body, mind, and spirit. You can combine conventional and integrative treatments—from medications and supplements to licensed practitioners—with an optimal diet and appropriate exercise to create an integrated plan of pain relief that best meets your needs.

Once again, my goal is to give you as much control as possible over the treatment of your own pain symptoms. One great way to start is to have a sensible diet that can keep inflammation levels down, leading in turn to less pain and fewer health issues.

PART II

SELF-CARE
(What You Can Do on Your Own)

Chapter Four

The Best Diet for You

One day toward the end of my medical training, I was meeting with my colleague Heidi Skolnik, who is a nutritionist on staff here at HSS. I wanted to discuss the possibility of having my patients whose overweight condition was making their arthritis considerably more painful receive nutritional counseling for weight loss. As we chatted about the obesity epidemic and the probable reasons behind it, Heidi educated me about the modern diet and how it can have a significantly negative impact on lifestyle disorders, including obesity, arthritis, heart disease, and cancer.

Heidi told me some startling facts about diet and nutrition that surprisingly few physicians know. During all my years in medical college, I received no clues about how drastically different the modern diet is compared to a diet only a hundred years ago. I realized that if we reverted to eating the kinds of food our immediate forebears had, we would be in much better health and have a far lower incidence of obesity as a nation. When I later spoke about this to my patient Belle, 56, who is overweight and who also has swelling and pain in the knee due to arthritis, she was a nonbeliever. But I persisted and asked her to give the diet a chance. After six weeks of adhering to an anti-inflammatory diet, avoiding fast food and processed food, she was astonished at how much the swelling in her knee had decreased. Like the majority of overweight individuals, Belle was taking in too much processed sugar in all its forms, along with simple carbs like bread and pasta that quickly break down into sugar. She was also deficient in the essential fatty acids known as omega-3 that keep cell membranes flexible and block the actions of some of the compounds that cause inflammation.

The sad truth is that all you have to do to set off an inflammatory response is to follow the standard American diet—eating readily available processed and fast food instead of natural sources of the proteins, carbohydrates, and good fats you need for robust health. It has been estimated that 90 percent of the food we in the United States purchase every year is processed and lacks essential vitamins, minerals, fiber, and antioxidants; in 1940, this statistic was only 10 percent. The number of people eating five servings of fruits and vegetables declined in the last 18 years from 42 percent to 26 percent. And 2,800 new types of snacks, candies, desserts, and ice creams are introduced to the marketplace every year.[1]

It may sound surprising that much of the food you can buy in your local supermarket can unleash the same response that the body would have to a life-threatening situation, but that is precisely the case—and I'm not just talking about junk food like candy and potato chips! Part of the reason for this development is that methods of food production have changed radically during the last century, so that the nature of the food we eat today is quite different from the food eaten not only by our ancestors, but even by our grandparents.

For centuries our ancestors have known that human health relied in large part on the food we consumed. As far back as the 5th century B.C.E., the Greek physician Hippocrates, considered the father of Western medicine, wrote, "Let your food be your medicine, and your medicine be your food." The overarching problem our ancestors faced, however, was finding enough food to stave off starvation, and avoiding poisonous or spoiled food that could cause serious illness or death. From the earliest days of prehistory, humans have been omnivores, consuming a combination of plant foods—including a surprisingly wide variety of fruits, vegetables, nuts, and berries—along with seafood and lean meats that were low in saturated fats. As hunter-gatherers, they ate what was available, and did not suffer from heart disease, cancer, and diabetes, the byproducts of our current poor eating habits and lack of exercise.

Of course, the average life span then was about 30 years, not long enough to develop many chronic illnesses. Most of the improvement in lifespan in the past two centuries has been the result of advances in sanitation and health care. Still, the United States ranks 42nd in longevity among modern nations. So why is this?

While some of this can be blamed on a lack of access to quality health care, the other most obvious cause is the fact that one in every three Americans is obese, and two in three are overweight. The epidemic of obesity can be only partly laid at the doorstep of our increasingly sedentary lives. Even people who do manual labor are becoming overweight because of the kind of food they eat, and changes in the way that food is produced. The plethora of diet books hasn't helped; if anything, the rate of obesity has increased in the last decade.

INFLAMMATION AND DIET

Research has shown that the everyday decisions you make regarding the kind and amount of food you consume have a significant impact on your health. Food provides more than energy for your body to function. It also contains vital nutrients, including vitamins and minerals that are critical for the well-being of your bones, and substances such as antioxidants and phytonutrients that can slow down the inflammation that plays a key role in the development of MSK pain.

The most recent scientific research has also found that nutrition has a direct impact on inflammation, which, as we have already seen, is one of the key components of chronic pain, osteoarthritis, and heart disease. Perhaps the most radical medical insight to come out of all the research into the relationship between food and its impact on the body is the role that certain foods play in initiating inflammation. Food and food additives that trigger inflammation are labeled as "pro-inflammatory" because they cause the body's natural defense system to respond in much the same way it would to a wound or other injury. For example, trans fats—a kind of unsaturated fat created by using hydrogenated oils—are known to increase the risk of a number of degenerative chronic ailments, including heart disease, diabetes, and stroke, by raising levels of "bad" LDL cholesterol and lowering levels of "good" HDL cholesterol. (LDL cholesterol transports cholesterol throughout your body and, at higher levels, accumulates in artery walls and makes them hard and narrow. HDL collects excess cholesterol and carries it to your liver.) Food manufacturers have known for a while now about the dangers caused by trans fats, but because trans fats enhance the taste of certain foods, as well as add calories and artificially slow spoilage, they continue to be used. This all adds up to higher profits for food companies, but the real costs of trans fats are shifted to consumers. Health authorities worldwide agree that we should reduce all consumption of trans fats to trace amounts.

Trans fats along with the preservative sodium nitrite, the flavor enhancer monosodium glutamate, sugar in its many forms (dextrose, sucrose, lactose, high fructose corn syrup), artificial chemical sweeteners, artificial colors, homogenized fats, and other toxic, disease-promoting ingredients, can still be found in abundance in the American food supply, all approved by the FDA.

These foods and additives promote inflammation by generating free radicals—atoms, molecules, or ions that lack an electron in their outer shell and seek to bond with other atoms or molecules to stabilize themselves. Once formed, these highly reactive radicals can start a chain reaction, like dominoes, forcing other molecules to become unstable in turn. They build up over time and cause cartilage to lose its ability to bounce back, artery walls to lose their ability to resist plaque, and airways to lose their tendency to remain open. The body reacts to inflammation in the arterial walls in a similar way to how it reacts to cuts and other external injuries. This can result in the formation of scar tissue that attracts plaque to artery walls.

Essential fatty acids (EFAs) are unsaturated fats that are called "essential" because our body cannot produce them, yet they are present in every living cell in the body and are critical for normal functioning of the body. The omega-3 EFAs that are found in foods such as cold-water fish (salmon, mackerel, sardines, herring, bass, swordfish, and tuna) and flax seeds, walnuts, and dark green leafy vegetables (including kale, spinach, chard, broccoli, and dark green lettuce) have been shown to discourage the production of inflammatory chemicals that harm the joints and other parts of the body. These omega-3 EFAs appear to turn off inflammatory reactions when the body no longer needs them, and so to keep the inflammation process from running amok. They also contribute to the creation of a variety of powerful anti-inflammatory substances.

By contrast, omega-6 EFAs, which are found in red meat and other animal products and in many vegetable oils used in cooking and baking, *promote* inflammation. Our diet is overloaded with omega-6 foods, including the omnipresent vegetable oils (corn, sunflower, safflower, peanut) not only used to fry foods and make potato and corn chips, but also added to most processed foods, commercial salad dressings, microwavable food, frozen food, and many brand-name breakfast bars and candy bars.

Until about a hundred years ago, our ancestors lived well on a diet in which omega-6 and omega-3 fatty acids were in balance. The ideal ratio of omega-6 to omega-3 fats is roughly 2:1, which has been our traditional diet for many thousands of years. Today, the ratio averages more than 20:1, which is dangerous to health. If you eat fast food more than four times per week, chances are your ratio is closer to 40:1. A study in the January 2002 *American Journal of Clinical Nutrition* determined that the omega-6 EFAs increased inflammation in heart cells.[2] Because omega-3 and omega-6 interact with each other, it's important to maintain the proper balance between them that is crucial for good health.

Belle, from the story at the beginning of this chapter, was a classic case of the problem that many people have today. Her lack of omega-3 intake coupled with excessive consumption of sugars had turned her body into a fat-making machine. Belle's lifestyle embodies the four key factors that I have become convinced are at the root of our obesity epidemic:

1. She takes in more calories each day than her body requires, and calories that aren't used are stored as fat.

2. She is lacking in sufficient omega-3 EFAs, which not only help decrease inflammation but also increase insulin sensitivity, making the body's cells more receptive to the insulin circulating in the body, thus lowering overall levels of insulin. Insulin is a potent hormone that is responsible for controlling the level of sugar in the blood. It triggers the cells of the body to use newly ingested food for energy, so having enough insulin in the blood makes sure that cells get the energy they need. But too much insulin circulating in the body makes it difficult to lose weight, because insulin also increases the activity of an enzyme known to increase the storage of fat. That's how insulin puts the weight on. For that reason it is essential to vastly increase your daily intake of omega-3 EFAs, which control insulin levels by as much as 50 percent, according to some studies.

3. She lives a sedentary lifestyle. General lack of exercise not only leads to fewer calories burned but also lower insulin sensitivity. A minimum of 30 minutes of daily aerobic exercise on most days of the week has been shown to increase insulin sensitivity.

4. Her intake of processed sugar is extremely high. Besides the processed sugar getting turned into fat, it also causes decreased insulin sensitivity and, so, higher levels of circulating insulin, causing weight gain and inability to lose weight.

These four problems have not only caused an obesity epidemic but have also led to an explosion in chronic pain, because obesity is linked to early onset of MSK diseases that cause chronic pain.

Through continuing conversations with the nutritionist Heidi Skolnick, and through my own reading and research, I became convinced that the less processed food we eat, the better. And that drastically reducing processed sugar intake, combined with increasing the amount of omega–3 EFAs in our diet, is essential not only for reducing pain but also for maintaining good health.

THE BASICS

Cathy is a 47-year-old occupational therapist who had been struggling with MS and hip dysplasia, a condition in which the femur doesn't fit properly into the hip socket. She was overweight, had already had two hip replacements, and was taking hydrocodone and NSAIDs. After following an anti-inflammatory diet by eliminating or minimizing sugar, red meat, and most dairy, she felt relief from the pain she'd been dealing with for years. But what really convinced her was what happened when she fell off the regimen—the pain came back, just as fierce as before. This was the beginning of her awareness of the power of food. Later, Cathy also chose to eliminate gluten altogether and lost a substantial amount of weight while eating mainly chicken, organic fish and other seafood, vegetables, and fruit. She was also able to stop using the narcotic painkillers she had been prescribed, and she cut down a great deal on the NSAIDs she was taking.

It's amazing that simply eating a healthy diet can have such a profound impact on your life. I now advise my patients to follow an anti-inflammatory diet, a variation of the Unified Dietary Guidelines that any healthy adult should follow to maintain health and prevent disease. In March 2005, the National Institutes of Health, the American Heart Association, the American Cancer Society, and the American Academy of Pediatrics created the guidelines to decrease the risk of life-threatening heart attacks, strokes, cancer, and other conditions. They recommend these daily limits for adults, based on a 2,000-calorie diet:

1. Total fat should ideally make up 25 percent of calories.

2. Saturated fat should be less than 10 percent of total calories.

3. Trans fats should be avoided altogether. If you can't give them up, then keep them as low as possible, less than one percent of total calories.

4. Lower your levels of "bad" cholesterol (low-density lipoprotein, or LDL).

The best way to follow these guidelines and maintain your weight is to eat primarily nutrient-rich foods that are relatively low in calories but extremely high in vitamins, minerals, and the other nutrients we need for optimum health, including protein. The dietary guidelines laid out below are designed to reduce the factors that cause inflammation and high levels of LDL, the "bad" cholesterol, by emphasizing plant foods, primarily fruits and vegetables, along with lean meats and seafood. High levels of LDL cholesterol, along with high levels of the inflammation marker C-Reactive Protein (CRP) are associated with heart disease, whereas high levels of HDL (the "good cholesterol") have a protective effect on the heart. You don't have to be suffering from chronic pain to want to gravitate to the foods that help fight inflammation. Indeed, if you are reading this book because a member of your family has chronic pain and you want to help, you can be confident that if you follow these nutritional guidelines and encourage your family to do likewise, you will be improving the length and quality of your own life as well as theirs. For example, eating five or more servings of fruits and vegetables each day will help reduce inflammation and related pain. But a study published in the June 2004 issue of *Archives of Ophthalmology* shows that eating three or more servings of fruit a day may also lower the risk of age-related macular degeneration, the primary cause of vision loss in older adults, by 36 percent compared to people who consume only one serving of fruit daily.[3]

COMMON SENSE AND YOUR DIET

Before we start discussing exactly which foods you should and shouldn't eat, let's talk a bit about the role of common sense in your food choices. It may well be that no one dietary regimen is going to be perfectly adaptable for everyone on the planet. The Mediterranean diet is based on what people eat in that region of the world, where the weather is warmer and they tend to lead more naturally active lives. They can probably get away with a certain amount of gluten in their pasta and bread. But if you're living in North America and you see that you're eating bagels and scones with your coffee, followed by breakfast cereal, a sandwich for lunch, and a pasta dinner with pie or cake for dessert, then common sense should tell you that you're eating far too many wheat- or grain-based foods.

Common sense also applies to portion size. A serving of any food is probably much smaller than you think. That may mean using restraint when defining a serving of meat or fish, but the good news is that it also means a piece of fruit or a small handful of blueberries, grapes, or raisins qualifies as a serving. The serving size of fruits recommended by the U.S. Department of Agriculture (USDA) is one medium-size piece—an apple, banana, kiwi, or pear; ½ cup chopped or loose fruit or ¾ cup of pure fruit juice, such as orange or grapefruit. For vegetables, a serving means one cup of leafy greens like kale or lettuce; ½ cup of denser veggies, such as peas or squash; or ¾ cup of vegetable juice. For grains, the standard is one ounce (one slice) of bread or cold cereal, such as granola, or ½ cup cooked cereal, rice, or pasta. When it comes to fish, poultry, or meat, a serving consists of three ounces, or about half the usual portion. Given the serving size for fruits and vegetables, five servings a day are not so difficult to consume. But your concept of a portion of meat or fish is probably larger than it should be. So if you eat a half-pound steak or six-ounce serving of salmon, consider that two servings rather than one.

To figure out good proportions, think of your dinner plate split into thirds: two-thirds of it should be plant-based foods, and the other third should contain fish, lean meat, or skinless poultry—all rich in the protein that is needed to build and maintain tissues.

Finally, common sense means respecting your own instincts and the value of dining as a source of pleasure and fulfillment. Instincts are not the same as impulses; you may have an impulsive desire to polish off a whole pint of ice cream when your instinct tells you it's a bad idea. If we pay attention to our instincts, they will usually lead us to healthful foods that are naturally delicious: fresh peaches and mangoes, orange juice, broccoli sautéed in olive oil and garlic, a green salad with fresh tomatoes, and so on. Now let's discuss the components of a healthy, anti-inflammatory diet.

WHAT TO EAT

Omega-3 Essential Fatty Acids

There are a number of different, helpful omega-3 essential fatty acids, and as mentioned above, they are found not only in cold-water fish, such as salmon, herring, tuna, anchovies, bluefish, and sardines, but also in flaxseed oil, walnuts, and dark green vegetables including collards, kale, and spinach. However, there are a few EFAs that are found only in certain sources. For example, alpha-linolenic acid (ALA) is found only in flaxseed oil, which can easily be added to salads or protein drinks or consumed by itself. The recommended daily dose for most people is at least 1,000 milligrams taken one to three times daily. Cold-water fish are the only abundant source of the two most effective omega-3 unsaturated fatty acids, known as eicosapentaenoic acid (EPA) and docosahexaenoic acid (DHA). These oils have been shown to reduce the risk of blood clotting, abnormal heart rhythms, and the creation of arterial plaque, and to be extremely effective in fighting inflammation. A study at the University of Washington showed that people who consumed two or more servings of fish rich in omega-3 each week were 40 percent less likely to develop arthritis later in life than those who didn't.[4] If you are unable to eat at least three or four servings of cold-water fish each week, you should be sure to take fish-oil supplements containing EPA and DHA. Later in Part II, I'll discuss this valuable supplement in more detail. But as with all supplements, they are meant to do just that—supplement your normal intake of essential nutrients in the form of whole food. So try to find more ways to get fish into your weekly menu.

When discussing the consumption of more fish, people often tend to have concerns about consuming too much methylmercury from deep-sea fish, but according to the Environmental Protection Agency this concern should be limited to women who may become pregnant, pregnant women, nursing mothers, and young children. In fact, the latest guidelines from the EPA are for the most part favorable toward eating fish, with the exception of the large predatory fish, including shark, swordfish, king mackerel, and tilefish, because they contain exceptionally high levels of mercury. They suggest eating up to 12 ounces a week of fish and shellfish that are lower in mercury, including shrimp, canned light tuna, salmon, pollock, and catfish. Albacore ("white") tuna has more mercury than canned light tuna, and so should be limited to no more than six ounces a week.[5]

Aside from being good sources of omega-3 EFAs, some shellfish are also helpful in fighting inflammation. Scallops are a good source of vitamin B12, which helps convert homocysteine into benign chemicals. High levels of homocysteine are associated with an increased risk of atherosclerosis, heart attack, and stroke, as well as with osteoporosis. Scallops also have good amounts of magnesium, which helps lower blood pressure (by relaxing blood vessels). And dieters have known for some time that shrimp are low in both calories and fat and yet are a good source of protein (as well as vitamins D and B12).

Healthy Meats

The reason most red meat produced in this country is so high in omega-6 is that most of our cattle are fed a diet of grains, including corn and soy, which are rich in omega-6. This is the result of another unfortunate recent development in the way our food is produced. In the early years of beef cattle production, cattle grazed on open pasture and ate grass. Remember all those western movies where the ranchers and sodbusters fought over control of the "range"—large stretches of grassland capable of feeding many head of cattle? In the last century or so, commercial beef producers figured out that if they feed their cattle grain as a food, production becomes cheaper and easier and requires a lot less land.

The problems that come from cattle housed in feedlots are twofold. The first problem is that cattle are not designed to eat grain. Their stomachs evolved to eat a diet of grass and green leafy vegetation. When cattle are fed grain, they absorb large amounts of pro-inflammatory omega-6 fatty acids present in corn, soy, and other grains. The second problem lies in the fact that the crowded and often inhumane conditions in which feedlot cattle are housed can increase their susceptibility to disease. The antibiotics used to contain diseases, along with the hormones used to fatten livestock even more, are all passed along to the consumer and further contribute to inflammation.

Meat from grass-fed beef, bison, lamb, and goats has less total fat, saturated fat, cholesterol, and calories than feedlot meat. It also has more vitamin E, beta-carotene, vitamin C, and health-promoting fats, including omega-3 fatty acids and conjugated linoleic acid, or CLA. In fact, pastured cattle have half the amount of saturated fat, and much less omega-6 than grain-fed cattle. And beef from grass-fed animals has two to six times more omega-3 fats than that from grain-fed animals.

Wild game, including venison and elk, are good sources of lean meat as well. Game birds, such as turkey, pheasant, and grouse are another alternative. Anything wild is more likely to be lean because it hasn't been fed grains to increase weight and purportedly to improve flavor, and has led a more active life. Some farmers who raise grass-fed stock acknowledge that they cannot graze their cattle and sheep year-round, and so have to feed them some grains, but far less than feedlot animals consume.

Dairy and Eggs

Nutritionists differ in their opinion of the healthfulness of dairy products. Some warn not only that dairy tends to increase cholesterol levels in the blood but also that the lactose in milk products, a form of sugar, can promote weight gain. They further believe that humans are not genetically disposed to process cow's milk and milk products including butter, cheese, and yogurt, because herding animals for their milk is a relatively recent development. But even proponents of paleolithic diets—diets based on what our hunter-gatherer ancestors are believed to have eaten as far back as 2.5 million years ago—acknowledge that our ancestors were likely to have eaten birds' eggs, and recent studies have shown that eggs do not substantially affect levels of cholesterol in most people. Indeed, they may actually reduce the risk of heart attack and stroke, because proteins in the egg's yolk help to prevent blood clots. A single egg also provides 11 percent of the daily requirement of protein yet contains only 68 calories. If you buy organic eggs produced by free-range chickens, you will avoid the negative effects of the antibiotics and hormones that producers of caged hens use. Some farmers now feed their hens grains that are rich in omega-3 to add another source of this valuable element to our diet. These eggs contain 100 to 200 milligrams of omega-3 (three to six times that of a normal egg). Hens that are allowed to graze naturally also eat a variety of grasses, and produce naturally healthy eggs. Their diets are supplemented by feed consisting of flax seeds that are rich in omega-3 fatty acids.

I strongly recommend avoiding or sharply reducing your consumption of all dairy and egg products except for eggs of the kind just noted. If you insist on consuming milk and related dairy, you'll be better off buying organic milk from grass-fed cattle, or yogurt and cheese made from the milk of sheep, goats, and buffalo, which are easier to digest and at least provide some calcium. Most organic yogurt contains the valuable *Lactobacillus acidophilus* bacteria that help us digest food (also known as probiotics). Eggs and dairy products from pastured (as opposed to grain-fed, feedlot-housed) animals offer you more "good" fats, and fewer "bad" fats. They are richer in antioxidants, including beta-carotene, and vitamins C and E, and they do not contain traces of added hormones, antibiotics, or other drugs. If you choose, you can replace the milk you normally use with the many milk-substitutes made from soy, rice, or almonds.

One sound alternative to yogurt, especially for those who are lactose intolerant, is kefir, a fermented milk drink that originated in the Caucasus region. It is prepared by inoculating cow, goat, or sheep's milk with kefir grains native to the Caucasus, but kefir will also ferment milk substitutes such as soy milk, rice milk, and coconut milk. Kefir has antioxidant properties, and contains a wider variety of bacteria that are friendly to the digestive tract, as well as lactase, the enzyme that breaks down lactose, the dominant sugar in milk. Some claim that kefir can also lower cholesterol levels or blood pressure, but these claims have not been proven.[6]

Vitamins and the Antioxidant Rainbow

Some vitamins seem to protect the body against inflammation while also providing us with many other benefits. The most important are vitamins C, D, and E:

- Vitamin C is the most abundant water-soluble antioxidant in the body; it repairs and builds collagen, the primary component of cartilage. You'll find it in citrus fruits and juices, green peppers, cabbage, spinach, broccoli, kale, cantaloupe, kiwi, and strawberries.

- Vitamin D (found in whole grains, dark green leafy vegetables, nuts and seeds, herring, eggs, milk, organ meats, and sweet potatoes) appears to help bones retain calcium so that they can absorb shock. Lack of vitamin D is the most common vitamin deficiency in North America.

- Vitamin E, the most abundant fat-soluble antioxidant in the body, helps shut off genes involved in inflammation and significantly reduces levels of C-reactive protein (CRP), which is considered a more reliable predictor of heart disease than total cholesterol levels. One of the most efficient chain-breaking antioxidants available, vitamin E defends against lipid peroxidation, a primary generator of free radicals. You can get it in its natural form from nuts, seeds, fish oils, whole grains, and apricots.

I mention the food sources of these vitamins because whole foods are a more reliable source of them than tablet or even liquid supplements. What whole foods have that many vitamin supplements lack is a wealth of vitamin-like antioxidant nutrients such as flavonoids and carotenoids, compounds that lend color to fruits and vegetables. A flavonoid such as quercetin, for example, is found in onions and apples and helps inhibit inflammation. The family of carotenoids includes beta-carotene, a powerful inflammation fighter found in carrots, apricots, squash, and other yellow-orange fruits and vegetables, but also in liver, egg yolk, spinach, broccoli, and yams. Whole foods contain complexes of these nutrients that appear to work more successfully in concert with each other than separately in extracted supplements. And so, it's important to eat as wide an array of healthful foods as possible. But, just as you can use fish oil capsules to complement your consumption of fresh fish, getting these valuable vitamins in pill form is better than not having them at all.

Fruits and vegetables that have the brightest, darkest, richest colors are the highest in carotenoids and bioflavonoids, the powerful antioxidants I just mentioned that help prevent inflammation. This means you can't go wrong eating lots of blueberries, blackberries, strawberries, red grapes, papayas, mangos, and kiwi fruit; dark green or red kale, Swiss chard, dandelion greens, beet greens, and spinach. It pays to eat foods of different colors from time to time, because pigmentation can indicate the presence of different nutrients. For example, one orange-red carotenoid (beta-cryptoxanthin) found in the highest amounts in like-colored foods, such as pumpkin, papaya, red bell peppers, tangerines, and peaches, may significantly lower the risk of developing lung cancer. Gourmet restaurants increasingly use unusually pigmented versions of staples, such as yellow beets, red carrots, purple potatoes, and rainbow chard to make their entrees more colorful, yet these variants often cost no more than the typical versions. So if brightly or unusually colored fruits and veggies catch your eye, indulge your sense of play and esthetic pleasure and try something new. I recommend that my patients eat at least five servings of fruits and vegetables a day, so varying the colors can make that more fun. And just remember if you need more motivation, these bright foods will not only help manage your arthritis and other MSK pain by combating inflammation, but will also reduce your risk of diabetes, heart disease, certain cancers, and obesity. What's not to like?

Gluten and Grains

Many healthful diets, including the Mediterranean diet, recommend eating a fair amount of grains, as long as they're whole grains, usually dark in color—brown rice or red quinoa, for instance. They claim that these provide a high-quality form of the fiber that we all need to stay healthy. Other diets, including several versions of the paleolithic diet, advise us to avoid all grains. The rationale behind the so-called paleodiets is that our forebears began eating grains only about 10,000 years ago with the advent of agriculture. Grain had several clear advantages: You could store it for those times when animal food and seafood were in short supply, especially during the colder seasons. And the grains themselves were the seeds needed to plant new crops. According to paleodiet theory, though, we are genetically conditioned to thrive on a varied combination of fresh fruits, vegetables, nuts, lean game meat, and seafood, and a few natural oils like flax seed, walnut, and olive, without resorting to grains.

The paleodiet has much to recommend it, although, like many recent diets, it has also attracted controversy. Some nutritionists question whether we really know what humans ate two million years ago; the diet's proponents, however, point to studies of the 80 or so contemporary hunter-gatherer tribes still thriving in various parts of the undeveloped world on just this kind of dietary regimen. Others question why we wouldn't have adapted to grains and agricultural staples over a period of 10,000 years. Most of the paleodietary recommendations overlap with those of the classic anti-inflammatory diet that I heartily recommend, however, and I have no problem with its basic formula. If you get most of your nourishment from a wide assortment of fresh fruits and veggies; selected nuts and oils; seafood (especially fatty deep-sea fish rich in omega-3); lean cuts of pasture-fed beef, and some wild game animals and birds, including free-range chicken and turkey (skinless breasts as opposed to dark meat), it's hard to see how you would either gain weight or set off an inflammatory cascade—unless you simply eat too much for your height and weight. And because protein tends to satiate your appetite, even that seems unlikely. You don't have to live without bagels, bread, pizza, croissants, cake, cereal (and all the other forms that grains can take), but cutting down on them will certainly help you keep your weight down, too.

And eating fewer grains, especially baked goods, might not be so bad. Grains do raise a number of potentially inflammatory concerns, in part because so many people have developed allergies to certain grains, especially wheat. Because wheat and products made with wheat flour are so commonplace in our diet, wheat allergies may cause inflammatory reactions even among people who are not aware that they are allergic.

Gluten—the composite of the proteins *gliadin* and *glutenin*—is the common name for the proteins in specific grains, including all forms of wheat (durum, semolina, spelt, kamut, einkorn, and faro) and related grains, such as rye, barley, and triticale. It shows up in many common food items from breakfast cereals, biscuits, and muffins to bread and pizza dough. Not all grains contain gluten, though, and those that are largely gluten-free include wild rice, corn, buckwheat, millet, amaranth, quinoa, oats, soybeans, and sunflower seeds.

Although gluten is a source of nutritional protein, it has some drawbacks. Some people have an intolerance to gluten, which can manifest in such ailments as celiac disease. Although celiac, a digestive disorder affecting both children and adults, is present in only about 1 in 133 people, its symptoms are serious. Your small intestine is lined with tiny, hair-like projections called *villi*, which absorb vitamins, minerals, and other nutrients from the food you eat. When people with celiac disease eat foods containing gluten, it creates an immune-mediated toxic reaction that causes damage to the villi. As a result, the villi are unable to absorb nutrients, which are flushed out with waste matter.

A larger percentage of the population, which isn't affected by celiac disease, can have an immune reaction to gliadin in gluten-based grains and their products, such as wheat flour. People with gluten sensitivity cannot properly digest gluten-based foods, and when gluten is undigested, your immune system interprets it as an invader that must be attacked. The immune system's attacks on gliadin can create large holes in the inside lining of the digestive tract, which may then be permeated and allow large gluten molecules to enter the blood stream. As the blood carries these molecules throughout your body, gluten molecules may settle anywhere and the immune system may then attack that part of the body. For this reason, people who are sensitive to gluten may suffer a wide range of illnesses far from the small intestine.

Beneficial Vegetables

As opposed to grains, beans and lentils provide an economical source of vegetable protein, complex carbohydrates, dietary fiber, and vitamins. Dried peas, beans, lentils and chickpeas are low in fat and good sources of iron, calcium, and minerals. Proponents of the paleodiet reject beans, lentils, potatoes, and tubers such as sweet potatoes and yams, because, they say, these are all toxic when uncooked, not all of the toxins are removed by cooking, and they were not eaten by our hunter-gatherer ancestors. This overlooks the fact that beans possess high amounts of soluble fiber that help reduce cholesterol. The high fiber content of beans and legumes also prevents blood sugar levels from rising rapidly after a meal, which makes them helpful for anyone with diabetes, insulin resistance, or hypoglycemia. All in all, beans and legumes offer a viable source of vegetable protein to balance your intake of animal protein.

Dietary Fiber

The last element of a healthy, anti-inflammatory diet that needs to be discussed is dietary fiber. Recent research has begun to suggest that sufficient dietary fiber may prevent cancer, diabetes, heart disease, and obesity, as well as many gastrointestinal problems. Fiber is an indigestible complex carbohydrate found in plants, rather than any single food or substance. Because your body can't absorb it, fiber has no caloric content. It also tends to fill the stomach and give you a feeling of satiation, so eating plenty of fiber is a great natural way to control your appetite.

The most valuable form of dietary fiber is insoluble fiber (cellulose, hemicellulose, and lingnin), which does not dissolve in water. Insoluble fiber helps promote regularity by adding bulk to waste matter and moving it through the colon more quickly and smoothly. This helps prevent constipation and may prevent colon cancer. Although fiber is not considered an essential nutrient, the Surgeon General and professional health organizations recommend a daily diet containing 20 to 35 grams of fiber—or about *twice* what the average American consumes. You get insoluble fiber from fruits, vegetables, beans, seeds, and whole grain products such as brown rice. Beans and lentils have the highest levels of fiber, followed by whole grains and vegetables. But if you have allergies to some grains or are wary of glutens and want to keep your weight down, fresh fruits and vegetables are your best bet. You can get the same amount of fiber (4 to 5 grams) from a large apple or artichoke as you can from two slices of whole grain bread or one cup of bran flake cereal. A cup of fresh or frozen raspberries has about 10 grams of fiber, and ¾ cup of broccoli is good for 7 grams, while a cup of spaghetti (whole wheat) has only 6 grams, and a medium bran muffin just 5.[7]

You can build your daily fiber intake by eating more complex carbohydrates—fruits, vegetables, and whole grains—as opposed to refined sugar and flour, processed food, and sodas. But increase your intake gradually over several weeks or you may experience diarrhea, gas, and bloating. As you eat more fiber, be sure to drink more water to help avoid gas. Once you get your intake to the desired level, you should experience no discomfort at all. You can use fiber supplements if necessary (*not* laxatives), but it's better to get dietary fiber from whole foods that are also rich in vitamins, minerals, and phytonutrients.

To get the most out of the protective, antioxidant qualities of all foods, you should eat a varied diet. Most people like to have different main courses throughout the week, but end up eating the same few fruits and vegetables (if they eat any at all). Certain foods are less expensive and taste better when they are in season and locally grown, and if you follow local and/or seasonal patterns, you'll naturally wind up eating more varieties of fruits and vegetables. Organic produce is more likely than crops grown by large agribusiness farms to have been cultivated in soil that isn't depleted of essential nutrients, and without the use of toxic pesticides, so they tend to contain higher levels of valuable nutrients and not be tainted.

Organic fruits and vegetables may also cost more and be harder to find, although most supermarkets now carry at least a small selection of organic products, including frozen fruits and vegetables with no added sugars or preservatives that are perfectly fine to eat.

In some cases, keeping frozen organic berries, broccoli, or stir-fry veggie mixes on hand causes less waste from spoilage. Unlike most commercial salad dressings, breakfast bars, fruit drinks, and other prepared items in grocery stores, the ones you'll find in health food stores are almost always free of partially hydrogenated oils, refined sugars, and chemical additives that promote inflammation. For example, many commercial brands of frozen fruits and vegetables add sugar, corn oil, or preservatives, so read the list of ingredients carefully.

For a quick overview of the good and bad food choices we've discussed in this chapter, consult the charts below.

Highly Recommended
Cold-water fish (salmon, tuna, mackerel, sardines, bass, anchovies); grass-fed red meat; free-range chicken and turkey
Flaxseed oil, olive oil, walnut oil, borage oil
Walnuts, macadamia nuts
Dark-green leafy vegetables, including kale, collards, spinach, chard, broccoli, bok choy
Cabbage, cauliflower, kohlrabi and other cruciferous vegetables
Fruits (apples, oranges, berries, bananas, papayas, grapes, kiwi fruit, mangos, avocados)
Whole grains (brown rice, oats, quinoa, but not wheat) in limited quantities if you tolerate them; beans and lentils.
Green tea, oolong tea, water, mineral water, 100% juice
Organic frozen fruits and vegetables with no added sugar (or anything else!)
Spices (ginger, turmeric, cayenne, garlic)
Dark chocolate with high cocoa content (70 percent or more)
Low-fat yogurt, goat's milk yogurt, kefir, coconut milk products, rice milk

Avoid or Minimize
Grain-fed red meat; feedlot-housed beef and chicken
Corn, safflower, sunflower, soy, and peanut oils
Peanuts; all salted, dry-roasted nuts; beer nuts
Commercial baked goods; all chips, pretzels, pizza; and other food made with hydrogenated oil
Deep-fried food
Chips, packaged snack food
Refined grain products, such as white bread, pasta, crackers, muffins, pizza dough, cookies
Carbonated drinks, juice drinks, soda, diet soda
Frozen foods with added sugar and preservatives
Most commercial, processed cereals; breakfast and energy bars; and salad dressings
Refined sugar, sweets (candy, cookies, cake, milk chocolate)
Full-fat dairy products, especially milk and cheese derived from grain-fed cows

Chapter Five

Exercise

When people suffer a joint or muscle injury, or begin to feel the acute pain of osteoarthritis, their first thought is often, "Oh, no, this means I'll have to stop working out! No more golf and tennis for a while!" They're afraid they may have to stop running, exercising, or doing yoga until their injury heals or the pain dissipates. But the truth is that it's essential to exercise to relieve pain caused by injury or arthritis. Proper exercise therapy can not only diminish pain but also significantly reduce the need for narcotic painkillers. And while helping decrease back pain caused by disc problems, for example, proper exercise can minimize the odds of those disc issues recurring. Some years ago, I had a series of revelatory conversations with my aunt, who had been suffering great pain from a slipped disc while she was pregnant. She told me that she went to see a yoga teacher, and that this master yogi gave her a simple yoga routine, which she demonstrated. As I watched her go through her routine, I began to see that there was much more that could be done for back pain that we were ignoring.

I became so convinced of the truth of this fact that I decided to design a clinical study to see if my perceptions were true for other people as well. I based the study on the same principles around which I built my first book, *Back Rx*. It was a randomized, controlled trial, which is the gold standard of clinical studies, and the results were conclusive. Patients who had been suffering from low-back pain for a minimum of three months and whose MRIs showed disc problems, such as a disc bulge, participated in my *Back Rx* exercise program for 15 minutes a day, three days a week. They also received the painkiller hydrocodone as needed and wore a lumbar cryobrace for 15 minutes before bedtime. A control group received the same medications and wore the brace but did not do the exercise program. After 12 months, 70 percent of the group that did the exercises reported over 50 percent pain reduction with good or better patient satisfaction, compared to 33 percent of the control group. The exercise group also took less time off from work and experienced a much lower rate of symptom recurrence. Those results were exciting, but what surprised me was that the exercisers also reported less overall use of painkillers even though they took more for the first three weeks.[1] Some of the exercises that were designed for this program can be found in Appendix B.

It's important to realize that if you are in chronic pain and undertaking an exercise program, you must first receive clearance from a physician. For the first few weeks of any new program, you may experience some increased discomfort, but in the long run you will reap numerous therapeutic benefits.

Exercising a minimum of 30 consecutive minutes on most days of the week has been shown to keep the cardiovascular system tuned up, which helps reduce or relieve pain in several ways. First, it makes the heart muscle more efficient, so that with each heartbeat you pump more blood. The reason your resting pulse rate goes down when you exercise regularly is that the heart doesn't need to beat as often to send the same amount of blood to the brain and the rest of your body. At the same time, this higher efficiency increases the ability of red blood cells to carry more oxygen. The net result of all that—the heart not having to work as hard, and more highly oxygenated blood reaching the brain and improving mental acuity—is that even moderate aerobic exercise controls pain and elevates your mood at the same time.

In addition, exercise has been shown to increase endorphin levels. The well-documented link between psychological and emotional stress and pain gives stress reduction an important role to play in healing most ailments and preventing their recurrence. The feelings of well-being generated by endorphin release help reduce stress and restore psychological balance. Persistent problems, such as MSK pain, disrupt the mind-body connection. Doing even moderate levels of exercise can greatly enhance your mental and physical balance. You not only become better able to bend without breaking physically, but you also grow more in tune with yourself mentally. You are better able to defuse stressful situations and reduce both physical and emotional tension before it accumulates to the danger point.

As mentioned previously, exercise also increases insulin sensitivity, thus lowering the level of circulating insulin in the body. With increased insulin sensitivity, it is easier to maintain or lose weight, and that can be crucial when dealing with chronic MSK pain. Clinical evidence has shown that daily exercise may also slow the progression of arthritis. Finally, our research has shown that a simple, well-designed exercise routine can minimize your dependence on narcotics along with lowering the recurrence of severe bouts of pain.

However, for exercise to be effective, it has to fit your individual situation. If you have shoulder tendonitis, you shouldn't be doing bench presses and pull-ups. You have to work around the pain to some extent, and learn how to use ice and heat to decrease pain beforehand and relax muscles afterward, as we'll see later in this chapter. But first, you need to know a little about the essential elements involved in proper exercise that will keep you pain-free—not only when you exercise but throughout your day.

THREE KEYS TO PHYSICAL HEALTH

When you think of physical health and pain-free ease, what images comes to mind? Maybe you see a polished athlete—a tennis player who can run hard and make an impossible backhand shot at the edge of the court, or a baseball player leaping high to snag a line drive. Or you might see a dancer who can bend down and sweep her hand across the stage, then in the same gliding movement pirouette in the air and balance on her toes.

But you don't have to be a professional basketball player or jazz drummer to call on the intricate arrangement of muscles, tendons, neurons, and fibers that make movement possible. Indeed, the simple act of walking requires thousands of minute balance corrections from a vast array of muscles and nerves just to propel yourself along at an easy gait. Not only do your feet have to move across the ground, but your hips, spine, arms, shoulders, and head all have to move in sync to maintain balance in your system. Some physical therapists even refer to walking as a form of controlled falling: As you move one foot forward, your knee bends to absorb the shock. Then your rear foot raises and passes the supporting leg just as your weight-bearing foot lifts off the ground at the heel and transfers the force to the ball of the foot. This is where your body starts to fall forward—and that free foot swings ahead just in time to meet the ground. If it didn't, you would probably crumple over in a messy heap, or end up looking like a character from Monty Python's "Ministry of Silly Walks."

Each of those carefully choreographed movements, which you've been doing for so long that they have become largely unconscious, requires the three key elements you also need to remain free of injury and pain: flexibility, strength, and endurance.

The first element you need to exercise and live without pain is flexibility, because a flexible body puts less tension on the muscle-tendon junctions throughout the body and makes you less likely to develop painful injuries. To remain flexible requires not only stretching and range-of-motion exercises but also adequate hydration. As we age, our tissues lose their water, like chewing gum that dries out and becomes inflexible. This dehydration affects the flow of electrical impulses that depend on water for relaying the signals that power our muscles and tendons. As we saw in Chapter One, pain signals are carried along a complex network of nerves made up of countless neurons that transmit electrical energy from various parts of the body to the brain and back again. A similar neuromuscular system of pathways carries a different set of signals through our muscle fibers, delivering and directing the electrical energy that allows athletes, dancers, pianists, and even airline pilots to perform at the peak of their abilities.

Loss of flexibility due to dehydration occurs not only in the muscle tissues but also for the fluid within our spinal discs, as I described in previous chapters. Instead of the "jelly dougnut" I talked about serving as a shock absorber between vertebrae, we end up with a stale cruller, shrunken and inflexible. Nothing can reverse this process, but you can certainly slow it down. The most important thing you can do, if you smoke, is to quit right away. The second key is to get down as close as you can to your optimal weight. And you should keep your body properly hydrated. That means drinking about ¼ ounce of water per day for every pound of body weight in cool weather, and ½ ounce in hot weather. So if you weigh 170 pounds, you'll need between 2½ and 5 quarts of water a day, depending on the season. You can count tea in that, as well as coffee. Contrary to popular belief, caffeine does not act as a diuretic when drunk in moderation, and does not cause dehydration or water-electrolyte imbalance. In fact, the most recent evidence suggests that caffeinated beverages contribute to the body's daily fluid requirements just as plain water does.[2] Fruit juice with no added sugar is all right, but too caloric to drink more than one quart a day if you need to control weight.

Along with flexibility, you also need the strength to balance and contain your movements—in both your extremities and your core. The core muscles that make up the trunk are called stabilizing muscles, and include the abdominals and muscles in the back. They are made of different kinds of fibers than the mobilizing muscles, such as biceps (upper arms) and quadriceps (front of thighs). The stabilizing core muscles, guided by the body's balance, need to be strong enough to allow the mobilizing muscles of the arms and legs to accelerate in kicking or swinging motions and then decelerate just as quickly without causing injuries. You may recall the story of John in Chapter One, who at age 14 injured his back when a wild karate kick missed its mark. He had strong mobilizing muscles in his legs that allowed him to make powerful whipsaw kicks. But the core muscles supporting his spine weren't strong or flexible enough to absorb an unexpected twist.

Remember that you need to develop strength alongside flexibility so that one isn't overemphasized at the expense of the other. We've all seen the results when bodybuilders work hard developing strength and body mass but don't do nearly enough to compensate with flexibility. They become muscle-bound: trapped by overdeveloped mobilizing muscles that make it difficult for them to execute simple bending movements and put them at high risk for muscle and tendon tears. But the good news is that you don't have to sacrifice flexibility to gain strength. Take a look at Olympic gymnasts in action and you see impressively muscular biceps and quads, then watch in awe as these athletes spin with speed and dexterity on the pommel horse or do full splits during the floor exercise event.

You don't have to work out for hours every day the way gymnasts and professional athletes do to gain that kind of strength and flexibility, but you do have to become aware of certain facts about aging. By the time you're 50 years old, you'll begin to lose about one percent of muscle mass a year. It's important to maintain your muscle mass before you reach that age, and to slow down the loss after that. Simple resistance exercises will accomplish much of what you need to do to maintain both flexibility and muscle mass.

The simplest basic exercise you need to perform, however, is walking a minimum of 30 consecutive minutes for most days of the week. If you cannot tolerate walking because of spinal stenosis or hip or knee arthritis, then ride a stationary bicycle or a recumbent bicycle with a straight back for the same minimum of 30 minutes at least five days a week, as recommended by the American College of Sports Medicine.

The third key element you need to remain free of injury and pain, along with flexibility and strength, is endurance. The only way to develop endurance is through aerobic exercise. About now you may be having horrible visions of torturous, hour-long sessions of high-impact aerobics, Tae Bo "cardio-boxing," and other endurance feats. Relax! If you already suffer from some form of chronic pain, that's the last thing you want or need to attempt. Even for healthy people in the prime of life, it's questionable whether training that way is useful for anything other than a career in professional sports. In fact, most scientific experiments regarding weight loss in conjunction with exercise programs have shown that moderate exercise doesn't help you lose weight any faster than simply following an appropriate diet. But those same levels of exercise—the minimum of 30 minutes of walking or bicycling five days a week—will help keep you from *adding* weight.

Balance

In Chapter One, I discussed the pain receptors that respond to painful or damaging stimuli, whose technical name is *nociceptors*. But your body is also home to a host of tiny cells called *proprioceptors*, an entirely different set of receptors found chiefly in muscles, tendons, joints, and the inner ear. Their job is to detect the motion or position of the body or a particular limb and feed that data to the brain in a constant stream. Your brain interprets the data about minute stimuli arising within the organism and uses that information to keep you physically balanced. If you want a graphic demonstration of this process, known as proprioception, just try this: Stand on one leg with both arms extended straight out to the sides at shoulder level. If you have even average sense of balance you'll feel fairly stable, with maybe a slight wobble. You can steady yourself further by staring at a point on the wall or the floor in front of you. The visual depth perception data are fed into your brain along with countless other inputs about weight, floor texture, and so forth. Now test your balance a little further by closing your eyes. You'll probably feel your foot and ankle making hundreds of tiny balance corrections moment to moment, but before long your wobble will worsen and you'll have to open your eyes and put your foot down to regain your balance. In the yoga posture called the tree pose (for details, see Appendix B), you challenge your sense of balance even further by resting the raised leg against the inside of the opposite calf or thigh, then put your hands together above your head. But as difficult as this pose is to maintain, you can become quite adept at holding it through regular practice.

Proprioception is what enabled you to hold that position even briefly with eyes closed. The better your balance, the longer you can remain steady. Balance is essential to body awareness, because it lets you know when your body is in proper alignment. It also helps you walk in a way that sends an ample flow of blood and oxygen to the discs in your spine, allowing them to breathe and remain supple. That's one reason why walking is such a valuable exercise, even though it may seem like you're not doing much because it's not strenuous. But "strenuous" isn't the point. Our ancestors spent most of their days walking or sitting on the ground for over two million years, and they didn't get arthritis of the hip or chronic fatigue syndrome. Sitting at a desk in a cramped position starves your discs of necessary oxygen, weakening your back muscles and reducing the ability of your hips to enjoy a good range of motion.

The main thing to remember about exercise is that, if done properly, it will restore the balance you need of flexibility, strength, and endurance, which form a dynamic triangle. Flexibility makes up the essential foundation for strength and endurance. A lack of flexibility creates increased risk of injury when working on developing strength and endurance. But you need to have all three elements in balance to function and live without pain.

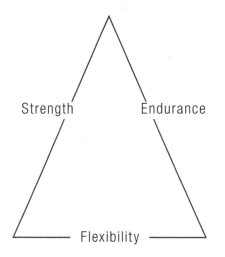

The key to all physical exercise is to learn from our ancestors, whose genetic structure we have inherited. As hunter-gatherers, they did far more physical labor than most of us, and had fitness levels shared today only by well-trained athletes, yet of necessity they alternated the kinds of exertions they performed. They might walk or jog long distances one or two days, then rest and do little for a day or more. Aerobic work might be combined with work requiring strength one day, or performed on different days. The 30-minute minimum walking should be considered just that, a minimum. There's no law saying you can't walk 45 to 60 minutes a day, six days a week. Or cross-train with weights a couple of days, and play a game of tennis, racquetball, or pickup basketball every so often. Exercise at moderate, sensible levels of exertion will not only help you maintain your weight and sleep better at night, but it will also help reduce pain for another reason: endorphins.

ENDORPHINS AND EXERCISE

You've probably heard about endorphins—the body's natural pain reliever—and how doing strenuous exercise can create a feeling of euphoria in athletes and ordinary folks alike. But even moderate levels of aerobic activity release endorphins in your brain, which mean exercise is important for pain reduction.

Endorphins do make you feel good, no question about it—that's why some people call them "nature's opioids" or speak of getting an "endorphin rush" after a hard workout. Indeed, the second part of the term *endorphin* is taken from *morphine*; the first part, "endo," is a short form of the word *endogenous*, meaning "internally produced." Taken as a whole, endorphins can be defined as morphine-like substances originating from within your own body. "Endorphins are neurotransmitters produced in the brain that reduce pain," says Dr. Alan Hirsch, neurological director of the Smell & Taste Treatment and Research Foundation in Chicago. "They have also been known to induce euphoria."[3] Narcotic drugs, including morphine, heroin, and cocaine, are classic endorphin releasers, but as we know, they can have horrific side effects, including addiction. Endorphins give you the high without the crash. So, what are they, actually?

Endorphins are compounds produced by the pituitary gland and hypothalamus during certain activities, including not only strenuous exercise but also excitement, orgasm, even laughter—anything that causes pleasure. Their resemblance to opiates stems from their capacity to produce analgesia (pain relief) and a sense of well-being. Along with sensations of euphoria and decreased feelings of pain, the secretion of endorphins leads to modulation of appetite, release of sex hormones, and enhancement of the immune response through their natural anti-inflammatory properties. With high endorphin production, the level of general body inflammation is lower and we feel less pain and fewer negative effects of stress.[4]

Another way of putting all this is to say that endorphins have natural antidepressant properties. To appreciate their value, you have only to compare endorphins with narcotics. For openers, endorphins decrease pain sensitivity, whereas narcotic drugs increase it. At the same time, endorphins increase the essential deep sleep called REM sleep, instead of decreasing it, as narcotics do—this is one reason why exercise helps you sleep better. Narcotics reduce intellectual acuity, whereas endorphins increase mental sharpness. And best of all, in contrast to both organic and synthetic opiate drugs, activation of the opiate receptors by the body's endorphins does not lead to addiction or dependence. In fact, consistent endorphin release can help reduce the need for painkilling drugs. Finally, unlike opiates, endorphins have inherent, natural anti-inflammatory properties that lead to decreased levels of inflammation in the body and, as a result, reduced pain sensitivity.

And now we have proof that the beneficial endorphin release from exercise lasts even longer than previously believed. "Moderate intensity aerobic exercise improves mood immediately, and those improvements can last up to 12 hours," concluded Dr. Jeremy Sibold, assistant professor of rehabilitation and movement science at the University of Vermont, Burlington, and lead researcher in a study presented at the 2009 meeting of the American College of Sports Medicine.[5] The mood of the exercisers was better than that of the sedentary group immediately after the workout and for up to 12 hours later, Dr. Sibold found.

"This goes a long way to show that even moderate aerobic exercise has the potential to mitigate the daily stress that results in your mood being disturbed," he said. What's more, men and women benefited equally, and the fitness level of the participant didn't seem to matter.

And you get all that from doing a little aerobic exercise several times a week, although, as I said, there are other ways to stimulate endorphin release.

- For many people, eating chili peppers leads to endorphin release, and the spicier the pepper, the more endorphins you release. Ironically, your body's protective response to the perceived "pain" of hot peppers is what triggers the release to help reduce that pain.

- Eating dark chocolate also leads to endorphin release, although, as we saw in Chapter Four, you need to eat the right kind of cocoa-derived, dark chocolate (and in moderation, one to three ounces at a sitting) to get the most benefit.

- Studies of acupuncture and massage therapy have shown that both techniques can stimulate endorphin secretion—and anyone who has had a full body massage knows it's hard not to feel good during and after receiving one.

- Sexual activity, especially orgasm, is a potent trigger for endorphin release.

- The practice of meditation can increase the amount of endorphins released in your body, as can certain other practices associated with spiritual traditions, such as chanting or communal singing. Religious faith is not required to obtain these benefits, but may add to them. Focusing on deep breathing patterns, which is similar to meditation, has also been shown to stimulate endorphin release.

- Experiencing the arts in any form, from art exhibitions to performances of music, dance, or theater, creates esthetic excitement that can release endorphins whose effects may linger as long as those from physiological release. Simply listening to music during a workout will help release extra endorphins, making the workout even more beneficial. It's what I consider the ultimate low-tech mind-body exercise.

- Excitement or danger of various sorts, from riding a roller coaster or sky-diving to hang-gliding or white-water rafting, can have positive effects. We tend to downplay the motives of "thrill seekers," but it's all relative to the nature of the thrill. As long as they're performed with regard to personal safety, these activities can reward you psychologically as well as physiologically.

Alcohol and Endorphins

The relationship of alcohol to endorphin release is a bit more complicated. Experiments in rats suggest that low to moderate amounts of alcohol release endorphins that produce a general feeling of well-being, but having just a bit too much to drink might reinforce the desire for excessive drinking, or trigger depression or feelings of desperation while actually inhibiting endorphin release. Christina Gianoulakis, Ph.D., a professor of psychiatry and physiology at McGill University and Douglas Mental Health University Institute in Montreal, and colleagues performed experiments using rats that yielded intriguing results. "Drinking low amounts of alcohol is associated with mild euphoria, decreased anxiety and a general feeling of well-being, while drinking high amounts of alcohol is associated with sedative, hypnotic effects and often with increased anxiety," Gianoulakis said, but she added a caution: "If after consumption of about two drinks of alcohol an individual does not experience the pleasant effects of alcohol, he or she should stop drinking." The problem, Gianoulakis said, is that researchers don't know the

---

mechanisms responsible for the fact "that some people can stop after one to two drinks while others cannot."[6]

One reason they can't agree on the positive values of moderate alcohol consumption is the very lack of specific research on human subjects. "The bottom line is there has not been a single study done on moderate alcohol consumption and mortality outcomes that is a 'gold standard' kind of study—the kind of randomized, controlled clinical trial that we would be required to have in order to approve a new pharmaceutical agent in this country," according to Dr. Tim Naimi, an epidemiologist with the Centers for Disease Control and Prevention.[7]

What's significant about those findings is that researchers have reached similar conclusions about the benefits of moderate alcohol consumption in helping to prevent heart disease and stroke. A drink or two a day seems to help, whereas more than that may cause physical or mental health problems, or both. So if you're one of those people who have trouble stopping after one or two drinks, you're better off finding other ways to stimulate endorphin release to help control pain sensitivity.

THE STOP PAIN EXERCISE REGIMEN

The following simple exercise regimen will provide you with all the physical activity you need to maintain basic health and work toward a pain-free life. It will also enhance your mind and body awareness so that your posture is well balanced and the mind-body system can operate optimally.

- Walking is one of the simplest and the best exercises that you can do to keep yourself pain-free. Walking is not only aerobic, which produces pain-relieving endorphins, but also weight-bearing, which helps maintain bone density and minimize the risk for osteoporosis. Walking should be done a minimum of 30 minutes consecutively most days of the week, at as brisk a pace as you can comfortably tolerate.

- If you have arthritis of lower limb joints or spinal stenosis that makes walking painful, riding a recumbent bicycle with straight back is a good option. My patient Howard is a 77-year-old executive who could not walk because of significant stenosis. He started on a program of bicycling daily for 30 minutes followed by icing his back. I told him that his enhanced ability to do the bicycle would translate into a better ability to walk. At first he was not diligent. After a little chat and some encouragement from his wife, he was on the bicycle every morning, followed by the ice. Within six weeks, Howard was able to walk six blocks without pain instead of two blocks. This illustrates not only the issue of proper exercise but also of compliance. Compliance is essential for self-care remedies for chronic pain. (Howard is now walking three times that distance with better balance. He receives a maximum of one or two epidurals per year, as opposed to the standard three injections he used to get before doing PT.)

- In addition to your walking or biking, make sure to take time on two to three days each week to stretch in an effort to maintain your flexibility. Some sports trainers devise elaborate, lengthy stretching routines to use before or after working out. Begin by stretching the major muscle groups, especially the hips and shoulders, always being careful to stretch slowly and smoothly, and not to bounce, which tends to tighten muscles. When the weather is cool you may need to warm up your muscles first with some light aerobic activity. If you participate in sports on the professional level or engage in high-risk outdoor activities such as rock climbing or mountaineering, you may want to devise your own routine. Just remember, stretching is helpful, but by itself hasn't been shown to prevent injury. And for most people with MSK pain, extensive stretching may do more harm than good, especially if someone is stretching you aggressively beyond the normal range of motion for a joint.

- Two or three times a week, also fit in strengthening workouts. Typical strength workouts can be as simple as 3 sets of 10 push-ups or modified push-ups (done from the knees).

- Take one day of rest and relaxation.

A Note on Breathing: When you're working out, always try to breathe in through the nose, out through the mouth. If you exercise strenuously, you'll eventually need to inhale through your mouth and nose together, but this is the best rule of thumb for low to moderate exercise.

RELIEVING PAIN THROUGH HEAT AND ICE

Even under the best of circumstances, you need to practice awareness when you undertake any exercise regimen. Simple walking requires that you be aware of the terrain, for instance; it may be more fun to walk in the woods or on mountain trails, but you're also more likely to slip and pull a muscle or twist an ankle on a rock or tree root. And it's helpful to stretch before and after a run or climb. But when you already suffer from chronic pain, you have to take further precautions, even if your most strenuous exercise is walking for 30 minutes on perfectly flat terrain. The best and easiest way to avoid or relieve pain is to learn how to use heat and cold to relax and soothe aching muscles and joints.

Indeed, the application of ice and heat remains one of the quickest and simplest methods of obtaining some immediate relief from MSK pain. My preferred treatment for chronic pain is to apply heat in the morning to relax muscles and joints that are stiff from a night's sleep and to increase the blood supply to the area. When you return home from a day's work or after any kind of physical activity—gardening, yard work, driving, traveling, or exercise—use ice to decrease the resulting inflammation and pain caused by exertion. Then return to using heat just before bedtime, to help relax muscles before the long night of rest. In essence, ice is the ultimate natural anti-inflammatory, and heat is the ultimate natural muscle relaxant.

One note of caution: Individual people may respond differently to ice and heat when used for pain control. Some of us simply prefer heat or ice at different times during the healing cycle, and you have to discover that for yourself.

Recent technology has improved on the traditional ice bag and electric heating pad with an assortment of products that are either reusable or disposable. But all of them are far more convenient than what was available just a few years ago. In an emergency, of course, you can throw some ice cubes in a resealable plastic bag, and that will do the job. But for regular, everyday use, it's hard to beat reusable gel packs that can be heated in hot water or the microwave, or cooled in a freezer. These gel packs are available in a range of sizes to fit your shoulder, elbow, ankle, knee, or back. Although they can be reused, you may still find it helpful to have a couple of each on hand so you don't have to wait to refreeze the same gel pack.

I also recommend several kinds of disposable pads that provide sustained heat that can help alleviate minor aches, pains, and stiffness in muscles and joints during the workday. (See Appendix C for specific brands.) They adhere to your body and are thin and flexible enough to wear under your clothes; they're also greaseless and odorless, so you can wear them at work without anyone noticing. Because these pads are disposable, they may end up costing more in the long run, but they are the most convenient option if you need relief at work or while traveling.

Chapter Six

Ergonomics

Ergonomics, simply put, is the scientific discipline concerned with designing the elements in your living and working environments according to actual human needs instead of appearance, comfort, or convention. The goal of sound ergonomic design is to do whatever is necessary to prevent repetitive strain injuries that can develop over time and can lead to long-term disability.

The principles of ergonomics apply to all areas of your life, not just the workplace. Because we tend to spend more of our time working than we do recreating, exercising, or even sleeping, it's natural to focus most of our attention on the conditions under which we work. But just as all areas of life are important to our happiness, they also can have an impact on our health and the levels of pain we may encounter. So, I'll begin by talking about significant workplace issues, but then give you some guidelines for avoiding pain in the rest of your life.

WORKPLACE ERGONOMICS

If you do manual labor of various kinds, work in a factory, or on an assembly line, you may have less control over your work environment than if you work in an office or at home. For most people who work at a desk with a computer, the rules are fairly simple but extremely important. Since our desk-and-computer-based situation is not going to change in the foreseeable future, we all need to practice common sense as we work at our computer screens and desks.

Choosing and Positioning Your Work Chair

Let's start with your chair. A number of fairly expensive ergonomic chairs have come on the market in the last few years, and there's nothing wrong with that. The Herman Miller Aeron, Mirra, and Backsaver office chairs are fine products, with prices ranging from $200 to over $1,000, although generic ergonomic chairs that look and function much the same are available online at lower cost. Pick the chair not by how it looks, but by how you feel in it. It should accommodate your body type well, have a medium-firm cushion or seat, and be height-adjustable, so that your thighs are parallel to the floor when you sit in it. Built-in lumbar support is a plus, but you can also get that benefit from a fasten-on lumbar support available at office supply stores and online.

The placement of your chair in relation to your work is also important. As you sit upright in the chair, you should be able to rest your elbows easily on the work surface with your forearms more or less parallel with the floor. Whether you are typing on a keyboard tray or working with a laptop computer on a desk or other surface, your forearms should have the same near parallel relationship to the floor. If your chair has adjustable armrests, fix them so they support your forearms in a position parallel to the floor.

In order to avoid exacerbating hip and knee arthritis symptoms when you sit, your chair should be high enough that your feet barely touch the ground. This prevents you from slipping back into a slouched position that takes your hips out of alignment and puts undue pressure on them. Think of how you probably sit when driving a car, typically very low with your hips slouched back against the seat and little to no lumbar support. That is why those with knee and hip arthritis have significant pain when they get out of a car and take those first few steps.

Good Sitting Posture

Even the best-designed chair cannot eliminate the effect of gravity and posture, so no matter what kind of chair you end up using, your posture in the chair should be erect, yet supple, with the top of your head, your ears, your shoulders, and your hips aligned, not rigidly, but more or less in the same flexible vertical plane. Your shoulders should not be hunched up or bent forward, as if they were attached to your neck. The shoulders are attached to the back, and they need to hang out easily behind and below your neck. When they do, your shoulders straighten and your neck muscles relax.

Finally, don't jut your jaw out and up. A poor computer setup can encourage this position, which strains your neck and back. It also constricts your breathing. Be especially careful if you wear eyeglasses, because you may have a tendency to bend forward or back to bring the computer screen into focus. Many people have a separate set of glasses designed specifically to work at the computer so as to avoid this problem. An optometrist can design a pair that's right for you. You will get better results by relaxing the back of your neck, making it long and straight so that you can look at the computer screen straight ahead or at a slight angle down. Your jaw should gently drop down a few fractions of an inch toward your chest, allowing the long cylinder of your windpipe to open easily. In this position you can breathe almost as fully and evenly sitting down in your chair as you can standing up.

If you have any experience of seated meditation, you may have already noticed that these same directions are often given by meditation teachers, whether you sit cross-legged on a cushion or on a standard chair. Precisely this kind of relaxed-yet-alert posture allows seasoned practitioners to sit in meditation for long periods of time. The idea, however, is not to try to sit permanently fixed in one alignment, as in some forms of meditation, but to establish the position you want your body to keep relaxing into, aided by good balance, as well as by core body flexibility, strength, and endurance.

But remember, the single most effective thing you can do to prevent desk work from injuring your back it to get out of your chair every 20 or 30 minutes to stand tall, arch backward, massage your spine with your thumbs, and, most of all, breathe fully and deeply through the nose for 30 to 40 seconds. This takes the pressure off the discs and lets them breathe.

An Ergonomic Workstation

Of course, there's more to good ergonomics than just a good chair and healthy posture. If you do a lot of typing or drafting at the computer, you need to be conscious of setting up that part of your workstation carefully. The computer monitor should be directly in front of your face, not off to one side, which will put undue pressure on your neck and shoulders. The top of the screen should be at eye level so that you don't have to bend your neck and head up or down. Keeping your neck level, use your eyes to scan down slightly, being alert not to hunch forward. The use of a footstool or swivel stool several inches high helps take the strain off the discs in your low back and your joints.

Improper positioning of the wrists can lead to carpal tunnel syndrome and other painful ailments. The carpal tunnel is a narrow, rigid passageway of ligament and bones at the base of the hand that surrounds the median nerve and tendons. According to the National Institute of Neurological Disorders and Stroke, if your tendons become irritated or other swelling narrows the carpal tunnel, the median nerve may be compressed. This can lead to pain, weakness, or numbness in the hand and wrist, radiating up the arm. As the condition worsens, many people report that their fingers feel swollen or tingling and they have difficulty gripping small objects or making a fist.

The best way to avoid this problem is to make sure that your hand and wrist are operating on the same plane. Get an ergonomic mouse pad that has a raised flexible support underneath the wrist. This will keep your wrist level with your hand and forearm as you use the mouse. You may also need to use one of the many newly designed ergonomic keyboards that help relieve "keying stress" that can lead to repetitive stress injuries. Bad ergonomics can put more pressure on your back, wrists, and shoulders, and even cause "tennis elbow" and rotator cuff impingement, two injuries that are usually associated with high-stress sports activities. When you throw one part of the body out of whack through repetitive motions, you start a whole "kinetic chain reaction" that can lead to serious ailments.

If you work while on the phone, then a headset is a must. Either wired or wireless (Bluetooth) headsets that connect to your cordless, desk, or cell phone allow you to use your computer or do other manual tasks while carrying on a conversation. These devices are inexpensive, especially compared to the cost of even a single doctor's visit, not to mention the pain that can result from holding the phone between neck and shoulder while typing. This arrangement also gives you the freedom to stand up and walk around, even to go to the kitchen and make yourself a cup of tea, while on the phone. Such changes will help to minimize neck problems. If you can help it, *never* hold the phone to your ear by bending your neck and pressing the side of your head against the phone and your shoulder.

Using a headset isn't only a matter of comfort or convenience, but also a way to do some of the standing and stretching I described earlier if you find yourself trapped in a lengthy call. (If you're on a conference call, you can even add some deep breathing. Just remember to push the "mute" button first!) Indeed, to make sure you stand up enough, try standing anytime you're on the phone for more than a minute. Standing tall allows you to breathe more deeply, is great for your back, and gives you heightened energy that will be heard on the other end of the line as persuasive, compelling confidence.

All of these suggestions for avoiding pain from the stress that's put on the spine in the seated position will work only, of course, if you remember to check your posture every 30 minutes or so. But in the midst of a busy workday, that may be easier said than done. For this reason I often recommend a standing workstation. Many people who have disc-associated back pain—specifically, pain that gets worse with sitting—could not have continued working without one. Solange is an active 38-year-old mother of two who has a chronic tear in her disc, leaving her unable to sit for long periods of time. Her back issues are manageable as long as she does not have to sit at work all day. Because Solange works for an international nonprofit, it took quite a bit of bureaucratic wrangling to get her company to pay for a standing workstation. But she finally won them over, and this workstation was the difference between Solange's being able to work comfortably (and then go home to take care of her two kids) and becoming disabled. In the end, paying for her disability would have probably cost the company more, so it was a classic win-win.

Standing workstations are really no harder to create than conventional seated stations. You can buy inexpensive standing workstations at many large retail chains, office furniture stores, or online, certainly for less than you might pay for a substantial wooden desk and ergonomic chair. The components of a standing workstation should be positioned in the same ergonomically sound way as a seated workstation—the difference is simply that everything is higher.

ERGONOMICS OUTSIDE THE WORKPLACE

The application of ergonomics outside of work can help you avoid injury when doing even the simplest household jobs or during recreation. Whenever you will be performing a repetitive physical task like shoveling snow or raking leaves, prepare yourself to do it safely by taking a few minutes to stand tall and do some deep breathing. Picture the motions you'll be making in your mind, and imagine yourself doing them in a graceful, easy rhythm. Every 20 minutes or so, take a break to reset both your breathing and your visualization. Just as when working at a desk, stand up tall, bend slightly backwards, and inhale deeply for a few moments. These steps will keep you focused and decrease your fatigue as you work.

Athletic Activity

Professional athletes spend a lot of time learning not only how to swing a bat, execute a forehand smash, or chip a golf ball out of a bunker and onto the green, but also how to visualize the proper technique. Even though you may be playing sports for relaxation and fun, you should invest at least some time in picturing yourself making the movements you would like to achieve. Always remember to breathe deeply and fully during these practice visualizations as well as when you are playing for real.

Be sure to use the proper gear at all times. If you run regularly, or even just occasionally, you need to use running shoes that are appropriate for your foot type. *Runner's World* magazine rates top-quality running shoes for each type of foot and has useful information about all kinds of footwear. One of the most common problems runners encounter is flat feet, so be careful to get shoes with excellent arch supports to minimize stress on your knees, hips, and back. Your feet are especially important for back health; any biomechanical weakness or imbalance will throw off the muscle chain that extends upward to your back. If you have any kind of misalignment in your feet, including fallen or high arches, you may need to get professionally designed orthotics to correct the imbalance. Don't buy shoe inserts over the counter, because they can actually make things worse. See a podiatrist and have your orthotics customized for your individual feet.

Obviously, the right sneakers are just as important for any athletic activity or sport, such as racquetball or tennis, which can put even more stress on your feet than running does. So if you're still using the same tennis shoes from five or six years ago, they probably won't provide the support and cushioning you need. And if you play racket sports, you also have to be conscious of the size and weight of the racket you use. If you have arthritis of the hand, be sure to use a slightly larger grip to minimize stresses on the hand and wrist.

Gardening and Yard Work

Spending time in your garden can be a great source of stress-reducing relaxation and reconnection with the earth that can lift your spirits and reduce depression—not to mention increasing your levels of vitamin D. But gardening can also place a lot of strain on your joints, especially your ankles, knees, and hips. Try not to stay on your knees for extended periods, or to bend forward as you plant and weed; use a stool and knee pads to minimize stress on the low back. As when you are at your desk or workstation, be sure to stand up and stretch at least every 20 or 30 minutes. Better yet, alternate sitting or squatting with standing positions at 30-minute intervals.

Fortunately, gardening gear has vastly improved in recent years, and you can now easily obtain useful items, such as padded kneelers with handles to help you lift yourself upright. Long-handled and telescoping tools allow you to reach borders easily without having to bend forward into positions that strain your hip and low-back muscles. These tools make it relatively easy to pull up weeds from an upright position without the bending and squatting. And many garden tools now come with a variety of detachable handles that let you choose the right handle length to make the tools height-appropriate.

In general, whether you're gardening or just doing basic yard work like raking, digging, mowing, and weeding, try to keep your work close to you so as to minimize reaching. Always avoid craning your head and neck in an extended position. Looking up while pruning tall bushes or trees for more than five minutes at a time, for instance, will create tremendous stress on your neck muscles and cervical vertebrae. Take short breaks every three to five minutes whenever your work requires looking up and extending your arms over shoulder level. And when you do work in that position, pull your shoulder blades together and avoid rounding your back.

In the Home

Many of the principles that apply when doing outdoor work also apply to indoor activities such as cleaning and cooking. Whether you're chopping veggies, vacuuming, or dusting, avoid craning your neck, overextending your arms, hunching your shoulders, reaching overhead for more than a couple of minutes at a time, and prolonged kneeling or squatting.

Kitchens are one of the places where you do a lot of work, which means they are also one of the places where you need to be most concerned about ergonomics. In older kitchens, ergonomics were not considered in design. Many have high cabinets that require straining to reach. Also, the traditional oven is an ergonomic disaster, making you bend to retrieve the heavy dishes that have been cooking. New waist-high ovens are becoming much more common.

If you are remodeling your kitchen, look into getting a separate cooktop and oven, so the stove can be raised. Also consider a raised dishwasher. This will mean that a part of your counter is higher than normal, but not having to bend over repeatedly to fill or empty the dishwasher can save you a lot of back pain. New refrigerators also are designed with ergonomics in mind with their freezer drawers on the bottom and the more often used refrigeration space on the top. You can also consider using drawers in place of some cabinets. Drawers allow you to get to all parts of the storage space without straining to reach behind things or being forced to remove everything to get the one item you need.

If you aren't currently in the market to remodel your kitchen, there are a number of things you can do in your current space to make it more ergonomic. If your counters are low and they cause you to hunch over when working on them, buy a thick chopping block that will raise the workspace. Also, be sure to arrange your kitchen so that things are within easy reach and heavy items are at waist level. Make sure to have a padded kitchen rug on the floor in any area where you do a lot of work—for example, in front of the sink where you wash the dishes. A rug provides relief from the pain and fatigue you may get from spending long hours standing on a hard surface.

Traveling

Going long distances, whether by car, bus, train, or plane, can be one of the most challenging activities for anyone with back pain. In the car, push your seat position as far back as possible so that you can extend your legs, and use a lumbar roll for your low back. As with gardening and housework, be sure to change your position every 30 minutes, and try to get out of the car and stretch every hour or so. Look for rest stations or service stations where you can safely pull over and really stretch your legs for a minute or more. If you're on a bus, train, or plane, try to get out of your seat and walk around every 30 to 60 minutes. When that isn't practical, at least check your posture to make sure you aren't slouching back in your seat. If you suffer from neck pain, you can now find excellent neck supports, and small lumbar supports and eye masks help for sleeping on long journeys. (See Appendix C.)

Sleep and Mattress Choice

One of the most significant elements in alleviating pain of all kinds, especially MSK pain, is getting enough good sleep. As you'll see when we discuss painkilling drugs, one of their worst side effects is the way narcotics interrupt your REM sleep. Because the body is designed to heal and regenerate itself during sleep, it's extremely important to get enough total sleep time, which for most adults means a minimum of seven to eight hours. If possible, finish eating at least three hours before you turn in, and never eat a large meal during that time period. If your body is using most of its energy to digest food, it won't be able to recuperate as well.

For good sleep, a medium-firm mattress is a good choice, although you may have to change it every three to five years. Better still is a 100 percent natural latex mattress, because latex, derived from the rubber tree, is a biodegradable material that is inherently antimicrobial, antibacterial, and free of dust mites. Latex inhibits the growth of mold, mildew, fungus, and bacteria, so it's ideal for anyone who suffers from allergies or asthma. Best of all, natural latex mattresses last much longer than standard mattresses, up to 30 years. Latex naturally adjusts to the contours of your body, providing orthopedic support that maintains proper spinal alignment without restricting capillary blood flow. These mattresses give just enough to be comfortable. Just be sure to get a mattress that is all natural latex, preferably natural Talalay latex, not a blend of natural and synthetic. But expect to pay for it—over $1,000 for a queen-size mattress. The brand name is less important than the assurance of 100 percent natural latex.

Futons are essentially equivalent to a medium-firm mattress, although some people find them harder. They are generally filled with cotton batting and/or foam and are much thinner than conventional mattresses. On the plus side, they rarely need to be replaced.

Ergonomically sound pillows can help align your back and neck in the same plane as they are when you are standing or sitting up. As a result, these pillows reduce stress and back pain and induce better sleep. Instead of tilting the head in an uncomfortable position, travel pillows allow the body and neck to stay straight and comfortable for long periods of time. Ergonomic pillows that help you get a good night's sleep are designed to support the neck and back; they usually have an indent in the middle and a bulge where the neck will lie.

If your bedroom is unusually light, you may also want to experiment with various sleep masks that eliminate all ambient light and allow you to sleep longer and more deeply. Be careful not to expose yourself to bright lights during the night—for example, if you get up to go to the toilet or to write down a dream—because bright light may signal your hormones that it's time to get up. Your body may stop releasing melatonin, a naturally occurring hormone that is important in regulating our circadian rhythms and helping to induce sleep. So leave a dim or blue night light on for bathroom trips, and keep a penlight next to your bed for dream recording.

Just as sitting correctly at your desk makes a difference in how you feel after a long workday, a good sleeping position will help you sleep well and feel rested after a night of sleep. Your best sleeping position is the one you find most comfortable and restful. Generally, though, sleeping on the right side puts less pressure on your heart, and sleeping in a modified fetal position with the knees slightly bent puts the least pressure on your spinal discs and low back. Sleeping on your back with a bolster or firm pillows under the knees also takes pressure off the low back. Sleeping on your stomach is the least ergonomic position. If you've always slept on your stomach, you may have trouble changing, but I don't recommend this position if you can avoid it.

Certain medications, including some antidepressants and muscle relaxants and most opioids, may disturb or shorten periods of REM sleep, during which we dream most actively. It's not a bad idea to keep a sleep journal to record what medications you have taken each night and how well you sleep and/or dream. The proper amount of REM sleep is not only needed to maintain a sharp mind and healthy body, but is also essential in managing chronic pain.

Remember that everything you put into your body, whether it's food, supplements, or medications, will affect your sleep in some way. Proper nutrition and supplementation should not disturb your sleep. If they do, they may not be right for you. In the next chapter we'll take a look at the nutritional supplements that I consider most effective in relieving and preventing pain.

Chapter Seven

Herbs and Supplements to Fight Inflammation

Anyone who grew up in the last century can be forgiven for believing that the best pain relief on earth comes in little white pills and tablets. Whether we take aspirin for a headache, Alka-Seltzer for an upset stomach, or ibuprofen for aching muscles, it has probably never occurred to many of us that natural remedies derived from plants and herbs can provide a similar level of pain relief. Better yet, these natural supplements have virtually none of the dangerous side effects of acetaminophen, ibuprofen, and countless other pharmaceutical drugs, whether available by prescription or over the counter (OTC). However, you should still check with your physician to make sure they do not interact adversely with any other medications you may be taking.

Some pharmaceutical companies make the claim that, because dietary supplements—a term that includes vitamins, enzymes, and herbal supplements—aren't regulated by the Food and Drug Administration, their safety and quality cannot be assured. In my opinion, lack of purity has been a big issue with supplements in general in the recent past. But in 2007 the FDA was granted authority to oversee the manufacturing of all domestic- and foreign-made dietary supplements. The regulations, which should be fully implemented by 2010, require manufacturers to follow certain "good manufacturing practices" (GMPs) to ensure that dietary supplements are processed consistently and meet quality standards of purity, strength, and composition—that they contain what their labels claim and are free of contaminants. Some herbal supplements, including stimulants such as ephedra and Ma Huang, can have undesirable side effects, especially if misused, and others may have an impact on surgery, so you should always let your physician know which supplements you are taking. But most of the supplements available in health food stores or online have been used safely for centuries, whereas pharmaceutical drugs are often put on the market after minimal testing, and have occasionally been recalled after they have proven harmful to a percentage of the people who use them.

If the idea of dietary supplements derived from herbs, fruits, or other plants to treat inflammation and chronic pain sounds a bit "New Age" to you, consider the case of aspirin. For many years, aspirin has been called a wonder drug with few negative side effects. (That view has been changing recently, however. Aspirin is almost never recommended over other analgesics or anti-inflammatories for severe muscle and joint pain, but it is still used as part of a regimen for heart health.) A brief look at the history of aspirin may help explain the way in which many other commercial drugs came to replace already existing natural remedies. In the 5th and 4th centuries B.C.E., Hippocrates was prescribing the bark and leaves of the willow tree to relieve pain and fever, including headaches, and this herbal remedy remained in use for more than 2,000 years. The active ingredient of willow bark was discovered by researchers in 19th-century Europe to be salicin, with which a number of chemists experimented to create salicylic acid. This medication helped reduce fever and pain, but caused severe irritation of the stomach and mouth. A French chemist named Charles Gerhardt mixed in another chemical to make it more palatable and called the compound acetylsalicylic acid; but he deemed the procedure too time- and labor-intensive to be commercially viable.

By the end of the century, Felix Hoffmann, a German chemist searching for ways to relieve his father's arthritis, studied Gerhardt's experiments, "rediscovered" acetylsalicylic acid, and developed an easier way to produce it. The company he worked for, Bayer, copyrighted Hoffmann's formulation and distributed it to physicians to give to their patients, first as a powder and later as water-soluble tablets, the first medication to be sold in this form. Bayer combined the "a" in acetyl chloride, the "spir" in *spiraea ulmaria*, the Latin name of the plant from which they derived salicylic acid, and the medical ending "in." By 1915 aspirin was available without a prescription. (Aspirin and heroin were originally trademarked by Bayer, but after World War I, as part of the Treaty of Versailles in 1919, the German company was forced to give up both trademarks.)

In 1948 California physician Lawrence Craven noticed that aspirin reduced the risk of heart attack in hundreds of his patients. Dr. Craven recommended that all his patients and colleagues take "an aspirin a day" to reduce heart disease. The American Medical Association now recommends taking a "baby aspirin" dose of 81 milligrams, instead of the standard 325 milligrams found in most tablets, to help thin the blood and lower the risk of heart attacks and strokes.

Although aspirin is still one of the most powerful anti-inflammatories and pain relievers, its use for that purpose has been mostly abandoned, because it poses risks of internal bleeding and stomach ulcers in the higher dosages required for anti-inflammatory and pain-relief effects, and safer natural alternatives are available to reduce pain in the body. Many other common pain relievers, such as ibuprofen and naproxen, known as non-steroidal anti-inflammatory drugs (NSAIDs), sold under a variety of brand names, offer high levels of anti-inflammatory and pain relief, without the very high risk of ulcers or bleeding associated with high-dose aspirin. But ibuprofen and naproxen and the modern COX-2 inhibitor celecoxib come with even more potentially dangerous side effects if taken regularly, including the potential for kidney failure, as I discussed in Chapter Eight. For that reason, you ought to try some of the safer natural anti-inflammatories first without resorting to pharmaceutical OTC products such as naproxen or ibuprofen.

THE HERBAL ALTERNATIVE

The good news is that a wide variety of herbal and vitamin supplements are known to reduce inflammation and can also help stop your pain as effectively as any of the commercial synthetic analgesics. These supplements are advantageous because they do not have the side effects that result from long-term use of NSAIDs, steroids, opioids, and other anti-inflammatory and painkilling drugs. Most supplements are at least as inexpensive as generic drugs and are readily available in most health food stores, some major drug stores, and, of course, over the Internet. Your worst dilemma in using supplements may be choosing from among the many brands, as there are still issues with purity, and which strengths will do the most to relieve your chronic pain. I will recommend dosages for each of the supplements listed, and in Appendix C I'll suggest a few companies that have proven most reliable and accountable.

In the meantime, let's take a closer look at some of nature's herbal bounty. As I mentioned, many of the supplements discussed below have been used for centuries to heal common ailments, long before synthetic medications were available. Because natural supplements cannot be trademarked or copyrighted, the major pharmaceutical companies have not helped to publicize them. Still, given the multibillion-dollar market for vitamins and supplements, some large companies have begun to manufacture and sell their own brands. As a sign of the increasing belief in their potential efficacy among members of the medical establishment, detailed studies on many supplements are being reported in mainstream medical and scientific journals. And top-tier medical institutions, including, for example, Memorial Sloan-Kettering Cancer Center and the National Institutes of Health, have begun to list detailed, carefully documented information about herbal remedies on their Websites.[1]

I've listed the following dietary supplements in order of importance, beginning with those that are most widely researched and acknowledged as effective in reducing inflammation and pain. If you need to refer back to the list for a specific supplement, you can quickly find it in the index at the back of this book. In some cases I've listed several options for obtaining a particular nutrient, any of which should suffice. Try one of these supplements at a time and see for yourself what results you get. If you don't notice any improvement within four weeks, or if you cannot tolerate a particular supplement, then try a different one or add another one. Having said that, I advise everyone to continue using some source of omega-3. If you can't tolerate fish oil, then use flaxseed oil. (Keep in mind that you can obtain some of these supplements by consuming certain amounts of the whole food or plant sources they're derived from, although that isn't always practical, given the amount you'd need to consume.)

THE BEST SUPPLEMENTS TO FIGHT INFLAMMATION AND RELIEVE PAIN

1. Omega-3 EFA: Fish oil (EPA/DHA), flax seed oil, green-lipped mussel oil

Dosage: 2,000 mg

We've already seen that the body needs omega-3 fatty acids—also called essential fatty acids, or EFAs—to function properly. Yet because the body cannot produce them, it has to obtain them from outside sources. If you find it difficult to consume sufficient quantities of fish or fish oil, a good alternative source of omega-3 is flaxseed oil or flax seed itself, both of which appear to be beneficial for heart disease, inflammatory bowel disease, arthritis, and other health conditions. (If you choose to eat flax seeds, be sure to grind them to a powder, or your body will be unable to absorb them.) Amazingly, one tablespoon of flaxseed oil contains more than 6 grams of omega-3, and 2 grams of omega-9, along with 1,800 milligrams of omega-6, a good ratio. Flaxseed oil also contains a group of compounds found in plants, called lignans, estrogen-like chemicals that act as antioxidants and may play a role in the prevention of cancer.

I recommend a minimum of 2,000 milligrams of either flaxseed oil or fish oil in vegetable gel caps. Be sure the brand of fish oil you buy specifies that it has been tested to be free of potentially harmful levels of contaminants such as mercury and PCBs and has the GMP stamp on the label. Another source of natural omega-3 is green-lipped mussel oil from New Zealand, which also contains high concentrations of glucosamine and chondroitin sulfate as well as vitamin B-complex, and has a good ratio of omega-6 to omega-3 EFAs. (See Appendix C for specific recommendations.)

If you like fine dining, extra virgin olive oil may be an even more appetizing source of natural anti-inflammatories. It contains oleocanthal, a natural organic compound that gives the oil its slightly peppery bite. The oleocanthal in extra virgin olive oil has been found to have anti-inflammatory and antioxidant properties similar to most NSAIDs. It has been proposed that long-term consumption of small quantities of olive oil may be responsible in part for the low incidence of heart disease associated with a Mediterranean diet. Olive oil is also rich in omega-9, which is technically not an essential fatty acid, because the body can make its own. While the omega-9 is beneficial, the real value of olive oil lies in the oleocanthal it contains.[2]

2. Ginger, turmeric

Dosage: 510 mg

Ginger (*Zingiber officinale*) is derived from a plant native to South Asia, and is one of the world's oldest, best-known, and most versatile medicinal foods. It has been used for centuries in massage oil in Japan and as a tea for coughs in China. It is one of the best natural anti-nausea agents available. When Indian researchers investigated their culture's ancient claims for ginger, they discovered that it did indeed relieve pain. In a 1992 study in which ginger was given to people who suffered from muscle pain, all of the participants showed at least some improvement. In the same study, the ginger treatment provided substantial relief for over 75 percent of those who had painful rheumatoid arthritis or osteoarthritis. And no participants experienced side effects, not even those who continued to take the supplement for more than two years. Ginger reduces inflammation, and thus pain, as effectively as ibuprofen and other NSAIDs, without their adverse side effects. It does this by partially blocking COX-2 enzymes, which are necessary for inflammation. Unlike synthetic NSAIDs, however, it does not block COX-1, thus it does not produce the gastric bleeding associated with those drugs.

Modern medicine is now recognizing some of ginger's time-honored virtues, especially for arthritis patients who want to decrease pain and protect their joints. The anti-inflammatory properties of ginger have been strongly supported by a number of scientific studies, including a year-long double blind study published in the November 2003 edition of *Osteoarthritis Cartilage*, in which participants who took ginger rather than a placebo experienced substantial relief from the pain and swelling of knee arthritis.

The potential of ginger to prevent nausea and vomiting after surgical operations and during chemotherapy treatment was demonstrated in a 1993 study in *Anaesthesia* on 120 patients for whom ginger was more effective than placebo and as effective as a conventional anti-emetic drug for preventing nausea after gynecological surgery, without that drug's adverse effects of drowsiness and depression. Carbonated drinks that contain high levels of natural ginger have been known to relieve common nausea resulting from upset stomach, morning sickness, and hangover.

Turmeric (*Curcuma longa*), a part of the ginger family, is also known as Indian saffron and jiang huang. It is an ancient culinary spice native to Southeast Asia that has been used as an anti-inflammatory agent for centuries in Ayurvedic medicine. Like ginger, the water-soluble curcuminoids in turmeric seem to inhibit joint inflammation. Turmeric has demonstrated anti-inflammatory and anticancer activities in lab studies; in one study with men who had surgery-related hernia, it reduced tenderness much more than the pharmaceutical drug some subjects were given. Like cayenne, curcumin contains pain relievers that stop certain neurotransmitters from sending pain signals to the brain. Curcumin has also been used to suppress inflammation in people with elevated values of CRP (C-Reactive Protein), which is now considered a significant indicator of risk for heart attacks and strokes. Bringing CRP values back to normal in these patients is believed to stop hardening of the arteries.

Turmeric is one of the main ingredients in curry powder, lending its characteristic yellow-orange color, and is used extensively in Indian cuisine. As a young child growing up in India, I saw the positive effects that taking natural ginger root had on my grandfather's arthritic knee. Ginger has mild blood thinning properties and may increase blood pressure if taken in dosages higher than 510 milligrams. You should check with your doctor before starting it, especially if you are on blood thinners or have high blood pressure.[3]

3. Glucosamine and chondroitin sulfate

Dosage: 1,500 mg/1,200 mg

Much has been made of the results of the Glucosamine/ chondroitin Arthritis Intervention Trial (GAIT), as reported in the *New England Journal of Medicine* in 2006. Test results of this high-grade clinical trial showed that "Glucosamine and chondroitin sulfate alone or in combination did not reduce pain effectively in the overall group of patients with osteoarthritis of the knee." The implication was that these nutritional supplements did not help relieve arthritis pain at all. What many media glossed over or failed to note at all was the report's *other* conclusion, which showed that "for patients with moderate to severe pain at baseline, the rate of response was significantly higher with combined therapy than with placebo." The report concluded, "Exploratory analyses suggest that the combination of glucosamine and chondroitin sulfate may be effective in the subgroup of patients with moderate to severe knee pain." That's a fairly impressive confirmation of the fact that these supplements worked better than prescription medication for people with high levels of pain, even though they did little for people with only "mild" pain symptoms. As the Arthritis Foundation summarized in its statement on the test results, "The more severe the pain, the better the response." Based on those findings, I feel comfortable continuing to recommend this combination of supplements.

Glucosamine and chondroitin are two molecules that make up the type of cartilage found within your joints. That cartilage undergoes a constant process of breakdown and repair, but if your body is going to repair its cartilage properly, it needs the building blocks to be available. Although there is no evidence that the glucosamine and chondroitin rebuild cartilage, they have been shown to provide significant pain relief, according to the GAIT trial. Further, the study on osteoarthritis progression prevention (STOPP), published in 2009, has shown that chondroitin sulfate may have cartilage-protective effects that can slow the arthritic process. In my opinion both supplements have natural anti-inflammatory properties that lead to their positive effects. [4]

4. Flavonoids

Dosage: grape seed extract, 500 to 1,000 mg

Flavonoids are a group of naturally occurring chemical compounds found in plants that act primarily as pigments. They occur abundantly in fruits and vegetables, to which they give their distinctive color; different flavonoids make blueberries blue, strawberries red, and summer squash yellow. Flavonoids (also called bioflavonoids, a term that is used interchangeably) are found as well in other foods, including coffee, tea, wine, beer, and dark chocolate. More than 4,000 flavonoid compounds have been characterized and classified, most of them commonly known for their antioxidant and protective activity. A number of studies have shown their unique role in protecting vitamin C in the body, which allows us to reap more benefits from this valuable vitamin. Studies from around the world support the fact that diets high in bioflavonoids are associated with lower incidences of most diseases.

Flavonoids are one of the hottest areas of research and conjecture in the world of supplements. Although they are often said to act as antioxidants, some researchers contend that the health benefits they provide against cancer and heart disease are apparently the result of other mechanisms. At the same time, a blend of natural ingredients from specific flavonoids, known as flavocoxid, has been made into a "medical food" that is available only by prescription. In a double-blind, randomized clinical study, flavocoxid was shown to have the same pain-relief effectiveness as naproxen, an NSAID, without any of the side effects. According to David A. McLain, MD, chief of rheumatology at Brookwood Medical Center in Birmingham, Alabama, "Flavocoxid is a good alternative to NSAIDs and COX-2 inhibitors."

Citrus fruits, well known for providing ample vitamin C, also supply flavonoids. Clinical trials have suggested that a combination of two flavonoids found in citrus may be helpful for treating hemorrhoids and beneficial for people who develop bruises or nosebleeds easily. These compounds are thought to work by strengthening the walls of blood vessels, and are widely used in Europe to treat diseases of the blood vessels and lymph system.

Grape seed extract contains flavonoids that have beneficial effects on the circulatory system, improving cardiovascular and eye health, and anti-inflammatory action. Results from animal and human studies including one at the University of California, Davis in 2006 show that grape seed extract may be useful in treating high blood pressure and cholesterol.[5]

5. Boswellia

Dosage: 200 mg

Also known as Indian frankincense because it is derived from the resin of a plant found primarily in two regions of India, boswellia (*Boswellia serrata*) has long been recognized in Ayurvedic medicine for its anti-inflammatory qualities that promote joint movement. It has traditionally been used to treat arthritis, ulcerative colitis, coughs, sores, snakebite, and asthma. Animal studies show that its major component, boswellic acid, has potent anti-inflammatory and antiarthritic effects; it inhibits joint swelling and pain associated with an inflammatory response. Scientists studying extracts of boswellia report that it can switch off pro-inflammatory mediators in the inflammatory cascade and reduce inflammation by blocking the lethal pro-inflammatory enzyme known as 5-LOX. Boswellic acid seems to have fewer of the adverse effects commonly found in steroids and NSAIDs, and long-term use does not lead to irritation or ulceration of the stomach, making it an attractive alternative.[6]

6. Bromelain

Dosage: 400 to 1,500 mg with 400 IU of vitamin E

Derived from the stem and juice of the pineapple, bromelain is not an herb but a mixture of sulfur-rich, protein-digesting enzymes called proteases. Pineapple has been used for centuries in Central and South America to treat indigestion and reduce inflammation. Bromelain, the bioactive ingredient of the pineapple, was first isolated in 1891 and is now approved by the German Commission E—a regulatory agency established by the German government to evaluate the usefulness of some 300 herbs—to treat swelling and inflammation following surgery, particularly sinus surgery. Although its primary uses are in the treatment of athletic injuries, indigestion, phlebitis, and sinusitis, and to help healing after surgery, doses of 200 milligrams have proven to be an effective alternative to NSAIDs.

Bromelain has been shown to have very good anti-inflammatory properties. In an extensive five-year study of more than 200 people experiencing inflammation as a result of surgery, traumatic injuries, and wounds, 75 percent of the participants showed good to excellent improvement, a substantially higher rate than that for NSAIDs or other drugs, and without side effects. Bromelain has also shown promise in the treatment of pain, numbness, tingling, aching, and carpal tunnel syndrome. Studies have shown that bromelain can reduce the clumping of platelets (which can lead to heart disease), the formation of blood clots and plaque build-up in the arteries.

More than 200 scientific papers have been written about bromelain since it was introduced as an anti-inflammatory enzyme in 1957, including evidence on its effectiveness in treating osteoarthritis. If you use bromelain as a digestive aid, it's best to take it with food. If you're using it for inflammatory conditions such as MSK pain, I recommend taking bromelain between meals on an empty stomach to maximize absorption. The German Commission E recommends 80 to 320 milligrams two or three times daily, but 1,500 milligrams daily is considered more effective for arthritis pain.[7]

7. Resveratrol

Dosage: 250 mg

Resveratrol is a plant compound found in the skins of red grapes, and in mulberries, spruce, eucalyptus, peanuts, and some Chinese herbs. It has antioxidant and anti-inflammatory properties and is believed to improve heart health. Resveratrol reduces the oxidation of low-density lipoproteins (LDL, the "bad" cholesterol) and inhibits blood platelets from adhering to the walls of arteries, which may prevent plaque formation and heart disease. It also acts as an anti-inflammatory agent with some positive benefits for managing chronic pain.

In 1991, a broadcast of the TV show *60 Minutes* popularized the so-called French paradox. It was known that although the French consumed much more saturated fat than Americans, they had at least 25 to 30 percent fewer deaths from coronary heart disease. The reason proposed by the program was the larger amounts of red wine drunk by the French, with correspondingly greater amounts of resveratrol. (The amount of fermentation time a wine spends in contact with grape skins helps determine its resveratrol content, and so white and rosé wines have much less of it.) Still, the concentration of resveratrol in wine seems too low to account for the so-called paradox.

An alternate theory claims that the natural saturated fats the French consume in the form of animal fat, butter, and cheese are more easily metabolized by the body than the unnatural saturated fats and trans fats that Americans consume as hydrogenated oil in processed and fast food. Still others point to the more relaxed pace of life in many parts of France, including the traditionally large, long midday meal followed by a light supper, which allows the body more time to digest the majority of its daily calorie intake.

Some researchers have now identified a particular group of polyphenols, known as procyanidins, that appear to provide even more protection to the cells of our blood vessels. Unlike resveratrol, procyanidins are present in wine at levels high enough to be significant. Further, clinical trials of grape seed extract have shown that 200 to 300 milligrams daily of procyanidins will lower blood pressure—an amount you can get from just 250 millileters of red wine (⅓ of a bottle). But, you could get considerably more procyanidin by eating an apple! The problem with all this is that observers became fixated on red wine rather than resveratrol itself. Not that wine is necessarily bad for you in moderation. The Mayo clinic reports research showing that resveratrol could be linked to a reduced risk of inflammation and blood clotting, but adds that it's not clear if resveratrol was responsible for the decreased inflammation.

Yet although resveratrol lacks clinical data based on studies involving humans, an unpublished study using rats showed that 250 milligrams of resveratrol can slow damage to organs by decreasing inflammation. It has no known side effects.[8]

8. MSM

Dosage: 1,000 to 2,000 mg, with vitamin C, 1,000 mg

MSM, short for methyl sulfonyl methane (METH-l-sul-FON-il-METH-ane), is found naturally in cow's milk, meat, seafood, fruits, and vegetables and is believed to deliver sulfur to the body in a usable way. Sulfur is a vital component of joints, cartilage, skin, hair, and nails and helps maintain the structure of connective tissue. In short, sulfur is critical to good joint health. MSM contains as much as 34 percent sulfur by weight. It's still not proven how the body absorbs the sulfur it needs from MSM, although preliminary studies in mice and horses suggest that it is incorporated into proteins and joint tissues.

After several reports that MSM helped arthritis in animal models, a double-blind, placebo-controlled study claimed that 1,500 milligrams daily can help relieve symptoms of knee osteoarthritis. Based on two double-blind studies of MSM for osteoarthritis of the knee, the generally recommended dosage is 1,500 to 6,000 milligrams per day, but I prefer sticking to the low end of those dosage suggestions. I have had many patients who swear by MSM, but in my opinion it still lacks strong clinical data.[9]

9. Vitamin D3

Dosage: 1,000 to 2,500 IU

Vitamin D plays an important role in the maintenance of organ systems, regulating calcium and phosphorus levels in the blood by promoting their absorption from food in the intestines, and by promoting reabsorption of calcium in the kidneys. It is also needed for bone growth and remodeling. The major forms of vitamin D are D2 and D3, of which D3 is the most potent. Vitamin D3 is significantly more efficient in raising serum levels of 25-hydroxyvitamin D—the hormonally active form of vitamin D that produces the most benefit.

Research is now beginning to realize the positive impact that vitamin D3 has on decreasing inflammation, leading to less pain. Vitamin D3 is produced when you expose your skin to sunlight, specifically ultraviolet B (UVB) radiation present in sunlight when the UV index is greater than 3. This level of light is available daily during the spring and summer seasons in temperate regions when the sun is highest in the sky, but less so in winter and fall. You need to spend only 10 to 15 minutes in the sun without sunscreen twice a week to generate adequate amounts of D3 through the skin of your face, arms, hands, or back. Too much UVB is one of the unfortunate side effects of climate change and can be dangerous, but too little can also be bad for your health. Tens of thousands of premature deaths are believed to occur in the United States annually from cancers caused by vitamin D deficiency. This deficiency can also result in poor absorption of calcium, which can lead to bone diseases. Lack of vitamin D is probably the most common vitamin deficiency in the U.S.. The *New England Journal of Medicine* has published research showing that a significant percentage of the population of northern states in the U.S., including the Northeast, have vitamin D deficiency. I ask my patients during their routine physicals to have their vitamin D levels checked.

We have long known that vitamin D3 is involved in bone health, but the latest research shows that D3 deficiency is linked to other health conditions, including depression and back pain. Researchers from the Peninsula Medical School, the University of Cambridge and the University of Michigan have identified a relationship between vitamin D and cognitive impairment in a large-scale study of older people. The study was based on data on almost 2,000 adults over the age of 65 who participated in the Health Survey for England in 2000 and whose levels of cognitive function were assessed. The study found that as levels of vitamin D went down, levels of cognitive impairment went up. Compared to those with optimum levels of vitamin D, those with the lowest levels were more than twice as likely to be cognitively impaired.

Vitamin D3 is the only vitamin the body can manufacture from sunlight, but because we spend so much time indoors under artificial lighting, and use sunscreens outdoors over concerns about skin cancer, we are underexposed. You can obtain more D3, especially during the colder weather, from oily fish, but some researchers recommend a supplement of at least 1,000 IU (international units), and as much as 2,500 to 5,000 IU.[10]

As I said at the beginning of this chapter, you can obtain some of these supplements by consuming the whole food or plant sources from which they are derived—but that isn't always practical. To get enough bromelain to relieve joint pain, for instance, you would have to eat quite a lot of pineapple. And, bromelain is most highly concentrated in the pineapple's stem, which is not nearly as tasty as the rest of the fruit! Nor would it be a good idea to keep drinking more red wine every day just to get extra resveratrol. And not everyone has the time to chop and blend fresh ginger into each of their daily meals (but if you do, don't peel it first—the highest concentration of ginger oil is in the peel).

Nonetheless, as is true of the phytonutrients in food, you may well obtain further benefits from the interaction of the many nutrients in a whole food, whether it's a filet of salmon, a handful of red grapes, or a slice of ginger. Since we have to eat anyway, we might as well take advantage of the nutrients in all the foods from which these dietary supplements are derived, but take them in supplement form as well to have a better chance of getting enough of the vital ingredients.

When combined with proper diet and exercise, along with many of the OTC pain-relief topical gels and creams available, these supplements form a synergistic system that can have a dramatic positive impact on managing chronic pain.

CHOOSING THE SUPPLEMENTS FOR YOU

As you try different brands and strengths of vitamins and other supplements, you may come to your own conclusions about quality. For a selection of brands that have been around for a while and conform to recognized standards of production, see Appendix C. Although they may not all say GMP on the label, their standards are at least that high. As a rule of thumb, don't bother buying vitamins or supplements in a chain drugstore or supermarket. They carry mostly corporate products that are generally inferior. Go to a reliable health food store or surf the net for trusted brands.

Some people prefer herbal supplements in tincture form—liquid extracts in grain neutral alcohol—instead of tablets or capsules. They point out that in the process of making tablets or capsules, the plant is first dried and then ground to a powder. Along the way, many of the plant's essential oils may be burned and lost. Tinctures are more rapidly and efficiently used by the body than tablets or capsules, because they do not have to be digested and absorbed in the stomach. Tinctures immediately find their way into the bloodstream on entering the mouth, and so the digestive system doesn't have to work to liberate the herbal ingredient from the fiber and cellulose in a capsule or tablet. A possible disadvantage may be that some people are sensitive or allergic to alcohol or choose to avoid it. In this case, you can dissipate the alcohol by putting the dose of tincture into an ounce of warm water for 20 to 30 minutes. Having said that, the amount of alcohol in any given dose of herbal tincture is minuscule, equivalent to that in certain pieces of ripe fruit. Most tinctured herbs tend to retain their medicinal properties longer than other preparations, because alcohol is an excellent preservative. When properly stored in tinted glass bottles in a cool, dark place, avoiding heat, sunlight, and exposure to air, tinctures will last for at least five years, compared to the average shelf life of herbal capsules (one year) or tablets (two years).

Chapter Eight

Conventional
Over-the-Counter
Medications

Through the years, I have had to help many patients who came to me with arthritis, bursitis, and other painful conditions that had already advanced beyond the beginning stages. I generally recommended that they consider following the regimen that has evolved into the one I'm presenting in this book. But I also took whatever other measures I deemed necessary to treat the intense pain and lack of mobility from which they were suffering. My general rule is always to begin with the most conservative steps first, before moving on to more advanced, risky, or invasive stages of care. In sticking to the age-old principle "first do no harm," I prescribe the safest combination of exercise and dietary supplements and topicals; if those don't get results, I may recommend the least dangerous oral medications. If those don't help, in turn, I would carefully prescribe other medications associated with a higher degree of risk. I might combine oral medications with some form of medical care that involved external physical manipulation, such as massage therapy, physical therapy, osteopathy, chiropractic, or aqua therapy.

Sometimes pain can be reduced or relieved entirely by the use of mechanical remedies such as orthotics—custom inserts in the shoe for foot or ankle pain—braces for the knee and back, or though the use of transcutaneous electrical nerve stimulation, commonly referred to as TENS, which involves the application of electrical current through the skin for pain control. I might also recommend that patients seek out psychotherapeutic help, including stress reduction and other mind-body techniques, because chronic pain can easily lead to depression.

Only if none of those courses of treatment bring the patient significant relief will I recommend various kinds of injections, minimally invasive procedures, and, as a last resort, invasive surgery. In Part III, I'll describe some of the varieties of integrative care, ranging from physical to psychological therapies, and in Part IV, I'll cover the most fruitful conventional medical options, starting with prescription medications. First, however, I want to show you the full range of OTC medications you can obtain without a prescription, the kind you can find in just about any drugstore.

ORAL ACETAMINOPHEN

Acetaminophen is known in other parts of the world as paracetamol. (Its most popular commercial brand name, Tylenol, is a contraction of para-acetylaminophenol). An analgesic (pain reliever) that was approved by the FDA over 50 years ago, acetaminophen reduces pain by elevating the pain threshold, requiring a greater amount of pain to develop before we feel it. It is a good first choice for those with moderate muscle or joint pain. Adults can take up to 1,000 milligrams three times a day. I caution patients to stay within this limit, because excessive amounts of acetaminophen can cause liver problems. While generally safe at recommended doses, acute overdoses can cause potentially fatal liver damage, and in rare individuals a normal dose can do the same; the risk is heightened by alcoholism. Acetaminophen toxicity is the foremost cause of acute liver failure in the Western world, and accounts for most drug overdoses in the United States, the United Kingdom, Australia, and New Zealand. You should take it with water 30 minutes before or two hours after meals. To minimize stomach upset, some people like to drink milk rather than water with acetaminophen. The drug takes effect in about a half hour; pain relief lasts about three to four hours.

Most commercial brands of acetaminophen also come in a timed-release form that contains 650 milligrams, so take only two tablets every eight hours. You should be careful to avoid taking other cold or flu remedies at the same time, because some of them contain acetaminophen, too, which can quickly exceed the recommended dosages. Like all drugs, acetaminophen has some disadvantages, including the possibility of side effects such as gastrointestinal distress, fatigue, and light-headedness. Like most of the medications discussed in this section, generic brands of acetaminophen are equally effective and generally cost less than the brand-name drug. Just be sure that the label lists acetaminophen as the primary ingredient. I generally don't recommend a daily dose of 3,000 milligrams for more than a week. I drop the dosage down to 2,000 milligrams after the first week of use.

ORAL NSAIDS

Nonsteroidal anti-inflammatory drugs (NSAIDs) include the traditional medications that have been used for decades to treat arthritis and other MSK pain. The term "nonsteroidal" is used to distinguish these drugs from steroids, which have a similar anti-inflammatory action combined with other, less desirable effects. The most prominent members of this group of drugs are ibuprofen and naproxen, which are all available over the counter. I don't include aspirin here, because, although it is an NSAID, I don't recommend using it at high doses for pain relief, due to the high risk of ulcers. I still remain a big believer in the preventive potential of low-dose (81 to 325 milligrams) aspirin when it comes to heart disease or stroke. I often suggest to my patients who have not responded to acetaminophen that they take ibuprofen, which works by decreasing inflammation and making the nerve less sensitive to pain impulses. For moderate pain, take 200 to 400 milligrams of ibuprofen every four to six hours. I recommend 1,600 milligrams maximum a day in order to avoid kidney problems and ulcers. For best results, ibuprofen should be taken with meals. Side effects are mild in most people and include abdominal pain, indigestion, and nausea. Once again, less expensive generic brands are readily available.

NSAIDs such as ibuprofen may cause ulcers, bleeding, or holes in the stomach or intestine. These drugs function by interfering with the action of cyclooxygenase-1 and -2 (COX-1 and -2), enzymes that produce prostaglandins, which send messages—both good and bad—to the immune system. Their messages trigger inflammation, but they also protect the stomach lining. So, while blocking these pain-causing messages is beneficial in the short term, if done for an extended period of time they put the stomach at risk. The FDA has acknowledged that these problems may develop at any time during treatment, may happen without warning symptoms, and may cause death. The risk may be higher for people who take NSAIDs for a long time, are older, or are in poor health, or who consume three or more alcoholic drinks per day while taking it. Indeed, it is best to avoid alcohol and cigarettes when taking NSAIDs, because alcohol and nicotine increase the risk of developing ulcers in the stomach or intestines.

Aspirin and ibuprofen have also been shown to accelerate the breakdown of cartilage in joints if taken over a long period of time. Although this breakdown of joint cartilage is well documented, few patients are ever told about it. This is another reason to take NSAIDs in short spurts to avoid complications in addition to risks to the kidneys and heart.

NSAIDs require careful monitoring when used by patients who take other medications, such as blood-thinning drugs, other NSAIDs, oral steroids, lithium, or methotrexate as part of their treatment for other conditions. Prolonged use of NSAIDs can cause kidney problems, especially in patients with diabetes. I almost never use NSAIDs for people with diabetes for more than two weeks, as they are at high risk for kidney complications. NSAIDs can also result in increased blood pressure. To avoid these complications during long-term use, I recommend "drug holidays"—no medications one day a week—along with blood tests to measure kidney function. You won't feel significantly worse skipping a day, because there is still enough medication in your system. Patients with diabetes should have these blood tests twice a year. Patients at risk for heart disease should have an annual blood test. In general, however, I advise patients to avoid long-term use of NSAIDs altogether and take these drugs only in spurts during acute pain stages.

Much of what I've just said about OTC NSAIDs such as ibuprofen and acetaminophen is also true for prescription NSAIDs, which we'll discuss in Chapter Twelve along with other prescription medications.

TRANSDERMAL HEAT PATCHES

As I pointed out in Chapter Five, heat is an effective pain-relief modality. Heating pads can be cumbersome, so I recommend using a good transdermal heat patch for pain relief, especially for those with chronic back pain or Achilles tendonosis. These patches provide a sustained six to eight hours of heat that has been shown to have pain-blocking effects.

TOPICAL ANALGESICS

Topical analgesic creams and ointments can be applied directly to the area that hurts. Because the medication enters the general circulation directly without having to pass through the stomach, these topicals tend to have few or no gastrointestinal effects from the drug itself. The delivery system also reduces peak levels of the drug, leading to fewer side effects. And avoiding a first pass through the liver, which may filter it, allows more of the drug to do its job.

A number of different medications are used in topical analgesic creams or ointments. Familiar brand names such as Capzasin-P, Menthacin, and Zostrix contain capsaicin, which works by reducing the levels of neurotransmitters involved in relaying pain impulses to the brain. Bengay and IcyHot are designed to help relieve joint pain commonly associated with arthritis. The menthol in these products works primarily as a local anesthetic for relieving pain. Aspercreme, Sportscreme, and other brands contain a version of salicylate, a chemical substance related to aspirin.

I'll have detailed information and guidance about prescription medications, including steroids, opioids, and narcotic patches in Chapter Twelve. But I hope you will take advantage of the other, safer options I'm offering in this book before considering prescription drugs, especially narcotics.

There has been a paucity of great OTC products for giving significant pain relief. Based on my experience practicing medicine, I strongly believe we need better clinically validated OTC options for people to take control of managing their own pain. It was this conviction that led me to form the Inflasoothe Group.

Now that you've seen the cutting edge of self-care options, let's take a look at how you can fully utilize all these options to manage pain arising from some of the most common chronic pain conditions.

Chapter Nine

Managing the 12 Most Common Pain Problems with the Stop Pain Regimen

The broad range of pain can make it a daunting subject to categorize—and to treat. From the minor but insistent throbbing of an average headache to the sudden, scary stab of a heart attack, the range of treatment options may be narrow or broad. Nonetheless, most doctors can usually agree on a remedy: simple aspirin or ibuprofen for the headache, a trip to the emergency room and ICU for the heart attack, followed by extensive postoperative procedures, medications, bed rest, and in many cases an overhaul of the patient's entire lifestyle.

For some of the most common chronic pain problems, however, there may be a wide range of options to choose from, in terms of self-care as well as physician assistance. These options are not all equally effective, and based on my years of practice I've developed a sure-fire approach to each common ailment that allows you a maximum of control, yet suggests when to also seek medical help and what kind of help will be most effective. The 12 pain problems I address in this chapter are representative of those I treat on a daily basis.

In the treatment plans I outline below, you should begin with a few assumptions. First of all, just about every one of these ailments will benefit from your following the kind of anti-inflammatory diet

I discussed in Chapter Four. Eating the foods I recommend while avoiding the pro-inflammatory foods listed there will tend to reduce the level of inflammation throughout your body. In many cases, especially if you control portion size and cut out sugar and most dairy and grains, you will be better able to maintain the best weight for you. Those two goals alone—not triggering the inflammatory response and keeping your weight down—will remove the most commonly debilitating influences on your health.

If you are currently taking blood thinners, you should check with your physician before taking any of the supplements or using any of the topicals described in this chapter.

Because the treatments I recommend here are based on my years of experience with thousands of patients, I have given the names of specific pain relief products that I generally prefer to use in my practice, including The MD System oil and cream that were developed by the Inflasoothe Group. But treatments also need to be calibrated to specific patients, and what works for one may not work for another. For fuller information about the products mentioned, along with alternative products that may work just as well for you, please refer to Appendix C.

In each of these treatment plans, I advise some form of exercise. As I said in Chapter Five, you don't have to wear yourself out with high-stress, high-impact exercises to achieve the overall benefits. Indeed, you may not be able to tolerate even moderate levels of exertion if you are suffering from some of these ailments. The key is to do just enough to build the muscle strength that will help prevent reinjuring yourself, while using enough stress to rebuild. For sample exercises targeting low-back and arthritis pain, please refer to Appendix B.

1. ARTHRITIS OF THE BIG TOE

This may sound like a funny place to begin, but the problem is more widespread than many people imagine, and the pain of an inflamed big toe is nothing to laugh at. As we get older, the arches in our feet tend to flatten out. This leads to excessive stress on the big toe, causing it to become arthritic and painful. The most effective self-care therapy begins with riding the stationary bicycle for at least 30 minutes, preferably daily but at least three days a week. Because the bike isn't a weight-bearing exercise, you won't be in danger of further inflaming the big toe.

On a daily basis you can apply Zostrix cream or The MD System strong oil in the morning and before bicycling. Ice the toe in the evening for 15 minutes, and take two capsules of Gingerflex twice a day (gingerflex.com), as the combination of ginger with glucosamine and condroitin sulfate will help alleviate the pain and inflammation. I have seen ginger exert a very positive impact on the small joints such as in a big toe. The best medical option is to get a custom-made orthotic from a podiatrist to help reposition your foot to take the excessive stress off the big toe.

2. TENDONITIS OF THE ACHILLES TENDON

To be more accurate, the proper medical term is *tendinosis*. Tendonitis implies that there is an inflammation (the *–itis* suffix) that needs to be alleviated, but the problem is actually a degenerative condition involving collagen breakdown caused by diminished blood supply to the Achilles tendon. Self-care options include using heel lifts of 1 to 2 cm (unlike orthotics, you should be able to find these in any good drug store or surgical supply store). Make sure you get the lifts for both feet in order to avoid imbalance. The heel lifts take pressure off the Achilles tendon.

In the morning, you can apply a small WellPatch, one brand of transdermal heat patch, to the heel to provide heat over several hours, either at work or while exercising. Once you remove the airtight packaging, these patches generate heat that continues for at least eight hours. (They are generally very safe, but be sure to follow the directions, and don't use a patch for more than eight hours in any 24-hour period on the same area. Obviously, if the pad gets uncomfortably hot, or your skin starts to feel irritated, remove it at once.) People with diabetes especially should check with their doctor before using a WellPatch around the Achilles tendon as they may have diminished sensation in that region. In the evening do 3 sets of 10 toe raises: stand on one leg, with your injured foot up, and flex your injured foot slowly up and down; follow that with 15 minutes of ice.

The most promising medical option consists of injections of platelet enriched plasma (also called platelet rich plasma, or PRP). This is a relatively new procedure in which the patient's own blood is used to extract concentrated amounts of platelets that contain a variety of growth factors. PRP is injected into the affected tendon under a proper guidance system, such as ultrasound imaging, to promote increased blood supply. I used this procedure with a 43-year-old runner who had a partial tear in her Achilles tendon and could not run due to pain for more than two years. Within three weeks she was essentially pain-free and was easing her way back into running.

3. MENISCAL TEAR

The meniscus is the cartilage in your knee that helps evenly distribute your body weight between the bones in your leg. When the meniscus is torn, your sense of balance is reduced, which may lead to more pain or cause the meniscus to get torn even more doing simple things like walking down the stairs. You can use balance exercises to help with healing of the tear and more importantly to reduce the chance of a re-tear, particularly by doing what's known in yoga as the tree pose. Stand on one leg with your eyes closed for about 10 seconds. Rest the sole of the opposite foot against the inside of the straight leg, or just let it hang loose if that's too difficult. Repeat five times every day. (If you're unable to maintain your balance this way, try standing on one foot with your eyes closed but with your hand lightly resting on a table or other sturdy object.)

Apply ice in the evening and Zostrix cream or The MD System strong oil in the morning. The vast majority of these tears don't require surgical intervention, but they do respond to physical therapy, especially the use of therapeutic ultrasound to heat the knee. Christine is a 33-year-old runner who came to me with a meniscal tear that was not healing despite physical therapy. Her doctor had recommended arthroscopic surgery. Upon inquiring what she did in physical therapy, I realized that she did not get therapeutic ultrasound therapy. I asked her to undergo eight treatments of therapeutic ultrasound over four weeks, because the deep heat from ultrasound increases the blood supply, helping heal the meniscus. After two weeks of ultrasound treatments, her pain had decreased over 70 percent.

4. ARTHRITIS OF THE KNEE

The best regimen is walking for 20 to 30 minutes (or, if you can't tolerate walking, then ride your bike) preferably daily but at least three times a week, combined with stretching (see Appendix B). Apply Zostrix cream or The MD System oil in the morning, and ice in the evening. Take a minimum of 2,000 milligrams of fish oil daily.

Acupuncture has been shown to reduce pain for knee arthritis done once a week, so I also recommend that. If those options fail, I offer patients injections of an artificial joint lubricant called hyaluronic acid. This lubricant has been shown to relieve pain for up to six months.

5. ARTHRITIS OF THE HIP

Again, I recommend walking or bicycling for 20 to 30 minutes at least three times a week, if not daily, and stretching (see Appendix B). The exercise I like for hip arthritis is to stand on one leg with hands on hips, and kick the other leg out to the side, in three sets of ten. Take 2,000 milligrams of fish oil along with 500 milligrams of the bioflavonoid Limbrel twice a day. (Limbrel is available by prescription only.)

On the medical front, the best option is massage therapy done once a week. Arthritis causes the hip flexor muscles to become shortened and massage helps to stretch and lengthen them, giving pain relief and minimizing the limp.

6. BACK AND/OR LEG PAIN FROM DISC BULGES

Part of the problem with all disc issues is that this area of your anatomy has a limited blood supply to begin with. Good blood flow helps most MSK ailments heal. Walking daily for a minimum of 30 minutes moves the discs up and down and improves circulation when combined with stretches (see Appendix B). Apply heat in the morning, then apply Celadrin cream or The MD System cream (if you have sensitive skin) or oil. If you don't get relief from the cream or oil, try plain, unscented WellPatches as described above for "Tendonitis of the Achilles tendon." But do not use the heat patches over Celadrin or The MD System cream or oil. You may, however, use Lidoderm patches on top of the cream. And get an ergonomically sound chair as described in Chapter Six.

The best medical option is a transforaminal epidural injection. In studies I conducted at HSS and published in *Spine Journal* in 2002, we had an 84 percent success rate for mostly sciatic pain caused by disc problems.[1] These special epidurals deliver a potent anti-inflammatory solution (a corticosteroid) to the junction of the disc and the nerve to eliminate the pain in most cases. When combined with the above exercise regimen, they have been shown to give long-lasting pain relief.

7. SPINAL STENOSIS

Ride a bicycle for minimum of 30 minutes preferably daily but at least three times a week instead of walking. Biking helps you maintain your strength and endurance without inflaming the joints or nerves in the back. You should follow the other instructions for back and leg pain caused by disc problems.

I also recommend radiofrequency denervation for all back pain caused by arthritic joints in the spine, because it has shown an 80 percent success rate in clinical trials.[2] This process heats the tiny nerves in the back via small needle-like probes and disrupts the pain pathways I described earlier. I have thousands of golfers in my practice who have been helped tremendously by this procedure.

8. ARTHRITIS OF THE NECK

Apply heat in the morning followed by Celadrin or The MD System cream (do not use the stronger oil on the neck), and ice in the evening. Get a special pillow for sleeping. I prefer a product called Wal-pil-o. If that doesn't help, try using a soft cervical collar with short end in front.

Here's a great exercise for neck arthritis. Stand with your back against a wall and your upper arms (elbow to shoulder) making contact with the wall and your forearms slightly raised. Then push into the wall with your elbows for a full minute, wait a moment and then repeat for another minute. This will stretch the front of your neck and strengthen the back of it

On the medical front, you can get facet joint injections into the arthritic joints, performed under fluoroscopic guidance, that are extremely effective for relieving pain. (Fluoroscopy is an imaging technique that provides real-time moving images of the internal structures of a patient using a fluoroscope, which consists of an X-ray source and fluorescent screen. The latest versions connect with an X-ray image intensifier and video camera that allow the images to be recorded and played on a monitor.)

9. ROTATOR CUFF TENDONITIS

The best exercise for this problem is called a capsule stretch. Lie on your back and stretch your right elbow across your chest and try to touch your left shoulder. Hold for one minute, pause, and then repeat. Repeat entire exercise on the other side. Once again, apply heat in morning followed by tiger balm or The MD System cream, and then ice in the evening. If this fails, the best medical option is a shoulder injection of cortisone, followed by physical therapy. If there is a full tear, surgical repair is the best option.

10. TENNIS ELBOW

A company called Aircast makes a "tennis elbow armband" with an air-filled cell and non-elastic strap. The "bubble" takes the pressure off the tendon, dissipating the pressure on the muscles of the forearm. Using this inexpensive device, do what are known as negative strength exercises: holding your wrist up, use the other hand to push the weak arm slowly toward the ground. Do three sets of ten and ice afterward. Negative exercises involve strengthening the muscle and tendon during the lengthening phase. This is the best way to strengthen the muscle-tendon junction.

On the medical side, *do not* get cortisone injections. Because tennis elbow is a form of tendinosis, as with Achilles tendinosis, the issue is a lack of blood supply. There is significant evidence that PRP (platelet rich plasma) has shown effectiveness in treating tennis elbow, according to the Stanford Medical Center trial published in 2006.[3] These treatments will work if you have only a partial tear of the tendon or no tear at all; if you have a full tear, then surgical intervention will probably be required.

11. WRIST JOINT PAIN

This ailment seems to affect many postmenopausal women and some older men. Take Gingerflex, two capsules twice a day since ginger has great impact on small joint arthritis. You can also apply a small WellPatch during the day. There are limited medical options with wrist joint pain, but one I've applied is an injection of hyaluronic acid (synthetic joint lubricant), although currently the use of hyaluronic acid for arthritis of the wrist is an off-label use (not as prescribed by the FDA). One of my patients, a 63-year-old lawyer who is an avid golfer, comes in every six months and gets one injection, and he has done very well with that treatment.

12. FIBROMYALGIA

As mentioned earlier, the most important aspect of treatment for fibromyalgia is aerobic exercise—a minimum of 30 minutes of walking daily. You should also take two grams of fish oil daily together with strict adherence to the anti-inflammatory diet. While this diet is important for dealing with all of these pain problems, it is especially helpful for fibromyalgia syndrome, because it helps keep your immune system at peak efficiency to combat the debilitating effects of this condition.

Medical options include biofeedback and a combination of Lexapro (antidepressant) and Lyrica (nerve membrane stabilizer). For some users, though, the side-effect profile for Lyrica, which includes drowsiness and dizziness, can be daunting. I usually have fibromyalgia patients walk early in the morning, as they tend to fatigue later in the day, and to take Lexapro in the morning and Lyrica at bedtime. Though you may have increased symptoms in the first two to three weeks, in the long run, daily aerobic exercise is one of the best therapies for fibromyalgia.

OPTIONAL HELP

If sticking to a routine is hard for you, you can turn to a number of external support systems for help. Simply asking a trusted friend or family member to inquire daily about your progress is a powerful tool for many people. You can also turn to the ever-popular personal journal to record what you did and when you did it. This is a method of self-regulation that works for some of my patients.

Other options are more technical. You can set aside time to create a system of reminders on your BlackBerry or other portable scheduling device you may carry with you on a regular basis. There are also professional services, such as mProCare, which, for a reasonable monthly charge, creates a customizable message platform that will allow the health-care professionals you work with to send text messages via cell phone that remind you of the various treatments for any given problem, including what to do and when to do it. For example, this system can prompt you to apply heat or ice, or take medications at certain times of the day. However, because mProCare is so new, there is not yet clinical data to support the efficacy of such a program. Data from programs in other countries clearly shows that receiving cell phone messages has helped with similar kinds of health-care issues, such as quitting smoking. For more information, please visit www.mobilepaincare.com.

PART III

INTEGRATIVE CARE

Chapter Ten

Physical Integrative Care

Just around the time I graduated from medical college, a landmark study on the use of complementary and alternative medicine (CAM) appeared in the *New England Journal of Medicine*. Led by David Eisenberg, the director of Complementary and Integrative Medical Therapies at Harvard University, the 1993 study showed that about one-third of adult Americans had used a CAM practice in the past year. Most of those who did so used unconventional therapy for chronic, as opposed to life threatening, medical conditions, including chronic pain. By 2005, a survey by the American Hospital Association found that 27 percent of hospitals in the United States offered CAM, up from 8 percent in 1998. Today, highly regarded medical centers such as the Mayo Clinic, Duke University Medical Center, and the University of California, San Francisco, offer acupuncture, massage, and other CAM services.[1]

Smaller medical practices also routinely offer a wide array of treatment options under one roof. Indeed, the very terms "complementary" and "alternative" are no longer even appropriate for treatments involving herbal medicine, acupuncture, massage, biofeedback, yoga, and stress reduction. Like many others who have embraced this wider range of treatment options, I prefer the term "integrative" medicine. Proponents of this style of medical treatment often refer to it as wholistic health, consciously adding a "w" to distinguish it from *holistic* health, a term that has become associated with an ever-expanding group of disparate therapies and techniques for symptom management without any clearly unifying identity. In either spelling, though, the term simply refers to treating the whole individual instead of merely one part or system of the body—in essence, treating the person rather than the illness through the many physical, psychological, emotional, and, often, spiritual networks contained within each of us.

At a time when health-care costs are rising astronomically, placing growing burdens on physicians' and caregivers' time and energy, this can only benefit both patient and doctor. To achieve the goal of genuinely integrative care, an increasing number of patients now work with teams of professionals from many disciplines. Besides general practice and specialist physicians who regularly treat arthritis and other MSK conditions, teams may include physical therapists, osteopaths, massage therapists, chiropractors, acupuncturists, nutritionists, naturopathic physicians, and psychotherapists. Mainstream health insurers are increasingly covering certain integrative treatments, such as acupuncture, which has shown positive results in treating chronic pain in many clinical trials, and the likelihood is that more integrative options will be covered in the future. Let's take a look at some of the most popular and widely accepted therapeutic modalities, integrative and otherwise.

PHYSICAL THERAPY

Because physical therapists receive rigorous training in conventional medicine and have extensive knowledge of the neuromusculoskeletal system, physicians are comfortable prescribing physical therapy. Physical therapists, or PTs, often begin by evaluating the range of motion of joints, a key factor in coming up with a treatment plan for MSK pain conditions, along with a variety of tests to determine muscle imbalances, flexibility, and other factors that enable them to tailor a program to the patient's specific needs. The physical therapy program may include exercises to preserve the use of joints, maintain strength in the surrounding muscles, and help the patient continue to take part in the activities of daily living. PTs also use a variety of modalities: heat and cold, aqua therapy, ultrasound (deep heat), electrical stimulation, and traction in conjunction with manual therapy and therapeutic exercises to achieve maximum results.

Although they can incorporate the results of laboratory and imaging studies, including sophisticated electrodiagnostic testing, such as electromyograms and nerve conduction velocity testing, most PTs work on a low-tech level that many people find appealing. What I find especially helpful about their approach is that they create stretching and strengthening regimes tailored to the specific areas of the body that are causing pain.

Physical therapists also use several devices to help arthritis patients cope with pain. For example, diathermy (electromagnetic waves of different frequencies) delivers heat deep into the tissues. They may also use the TENS units mentioned in Chapter Eight. These devices, which consist of a battery pack and electrodes and are usually connected to the skin, produce a pleasant tingling sensation and have been remarkably successful in relieving a wide range of pain and discomfort.

Physical therapists can suggest assistive devices to make it easier to perform household chores and activities at work, such as long-handled grippers designed to grasp and replace out-of-reach objects. They can also teach patients how to use proper body mechanics to get in and out of cars, chairs, or bathtubs, or how to lift objects to minimize stress on joints. Physical therapy can take place at a hospital or in a patient's home. Those who have completed the orthopedic specialty certificate or hold a doctorate in physical therapy are a good choice.

As in any profession, the quality of PTs can vary quite a bit. Over ten years of practice in New York, I have put together a network of seasoned therapists who have outstanding manual skills. I refer most of my patients to PTs as a trial or after undergoing minimally invasive procedures. Howard is a 77-year-old business executive who used to come to me for an epidural injection every four months to relieve the pain from his spinal stenosis. I finally convinced him to give physical therapy a try. He complained that he did not have the time and did not believe that it would benefit him. After persistent lobbying on my part, Howard started seeing a PT twice a week. After eight weeks, his gait, balance, and posture had improved dramatically—so much so that he now needed the injections at most every six months. I have repeatedly seen firsthand the positive impact of good physical therapy for chronic conditions such as spinal stenosis and hip or knee arthritis. Therapists must possess excellent manual skills and knowledge of proper therapeutic exercises for each condition.

OSTEOPATHY

In addition to physical therapists, you can avail yourself of the services of other professionals, such as osteopaths, who provide body-based procedures. Osteopaths believe that the body has self-healing mechanisms and that one way to release them is by therapeutic manipulation of the bones, joints, and soft tissues. Therapeutic manipulation of the body has ancient roots: Hippocrates used it in the 5th century B.C.E., but it was not until the birth of osteopathy in the 1890s that formalized programs were developed. Today, osteopathic medical schools provide rigorous education in the basic sciences as well as all aspects of human health, similar to conventional medical schools. Osteopaths learn to use their hands to identify the areas where the patient is experiencing pain. Then they apply one or more of 30 different manual techniques to restore the disordered body framework to optimal mechanical and structural ease.

The goal is to enhance overall bodily movement, along with the function of the nervous and circulatory systems, and to improve nutrition and drainage to tissues by way of assisting the body's healing processes. I recently saw an 18-year-old student from Turkey who looked like he had a significant leg length discrepancy. Upon examining him, I realized that he did not really have a genuine discrepancy in leg length, but a condition osteopaths call pelvic torsion. I sent him to one of the premier osteopaths in the country, and within two sessions of osteopathic treatments, the student's leg length discrepancy that limited his ability to walk properly had resolved by over 80 percent.

CHIROPRACTIC

Chiropractors give special attention to the physiological and biochemical aspects of the body, "including structural, spinal, musculoskeletal, neurological, vascular, nutritional, emotional, and environmental relationships," according to the American Chiropractic Association. The practice and procedures that chiropractors employ include adjustment and manipulation of the joints and adjacent tissues, particularly the spinal column. Chiropractic is a drug-free, nonsurgical science, so chiropractors don't prescribe pharmaceuticals or invasive surgery.

The roots of chiropractic care can be traced back to China and Greece in the second and third millennia b.c.e. Hippocrates published texts describing the importance of chiropractic care, writing, "Get knowledge of the spine, for this is the requisite for many diseases." In this country, the practice of spinal manipulation began to gain acceptance during the late 19th century. Daniel David Palmer founded chiropractic in 1895 in Davenport, Iowa, and defined it as "a science of healing without drugs." Traditionally, chiropractors assume that a spinal joint dysfunction interferes with the body's function and needs to be "adjusted" to return the patient to health. For many years, this notion brought ridicule from mainstream science and conventional medicine. Today, though, many doctors are comfortable sending patients to chiropractors to help treat specific conditions.

Some practitioners emphasize the "innate intelligence" of the body and spinal adjustments, meaning that the body knows how to heal itself with minimal help from practitioners. Still, the majority of chiropractors today are open to both conventional and integrative medical techniques, such as exercise, massage, nutritional supplements, and acupuncture. Although there have been numerous trials of manipulative therapy for back-pain patients, few studies of its effectiveness in treating arthritis have been undertaken. Nonetheless, I have seen my patients with lower-back arthritis benefit greatly from gentle chiropractic manipulations. Accredited chiropractors have the initials D.C., for Doctor of Chiropractic, after their name. I caution patients with neck arthritis to avoid aggressive manipulations, because they may be at risk for stroke or spinal cord injuries, although many chiropractors might disagree with me. For patients who have acute back pain or flare-up of chronic pain, chiropractic treatments are of tremendous benefit.[2]

MASSAGE THERAPY

Massage is one of the oldest healing arts, dating back at least 3,000 years in China, and is found among records left by the ancient Hindus, Persians, and Egyptians. Hippocrates, who seems to have documented so many elements of today's medical data bank, from the key ingredient in aspirin to the importance of a healthy diet, wrote papers recommending the use of friction for joint and circulatory issues. The word *massage* itself has been traced to French, Greek, and Arabic roots, but one intriguing source that has been suggested is the Hebrew *me-sakj* "to anoint with oil," which is the same root from which the word *messiah* comes. If you've ever had a good professional massage, you may feel like salvation from your pains and anxieties is indeed at hand! Because stress is widely regarded as being responsible for up to 80 percent of physical ailments, anything that can reduce stress is bound to help alleviate pain and suffering.

Medical massage can be an important component of many patients' treatment plans. During a massage, a therapist manipulates the body's soft tissues—the muscles, skin, and tendons—using fingertips, hands, and fists. Massage therapists, as well as physical therapists, can perform massages, of which there are several types. Swedish is the most common form, and the first to become popular in the United States, introduced in the mid-1800s by two New York physicians; it is based on techniques developed in Sweden. This kind of massage consists of long, smooth strokes and kneading movements along the skin. All parts of the body can be worked during Swedish massage.

But other forms of deep tissue massage have become increasingly popular in recent years. "Unlike Swedish massage, which concentrates on the soft tissues near the surface of the skin," says Rick Sharpell, a talented massage therapist in New York, "deep massage uses slow, heavy strokes to create direct pressure and friction on the muscles. The target of this massage is the deep muscle tissue. Some massage therapists combine these techniques to help patients [achieve relief] with specific muscle groups."

Therapeutic massage has slowly won the approval of a growing number of physicians, and therapies provided as part of a treatment prescribed by a doctor or registered physical therapist are often covered by mainstream insurance providers. The *Annals of Internal Medicine* published a study in 2003 showing that massage therapy is as good as NSAIDs for pain relief, but it needs to be performed at least once a week.[3] I have also seen good results from massage therapy for hip arthritis. If you can afford the added expense or if it is covered by your provider, you should try incorporating massage into your treatment plan.

ACUPUNCTURE AND ACUPRESSURE

Acupuncture has become one of the most popular therapies in the United States. The National Institutes of Health estimates that more than 15 million individuals in this country have tried the therapy for conditions ranging from arthritis and asthma to nausea and chronic pain. The practice of inserting ultra-thin needles into specific body points to improve health and well-being, and to relieve pain or for therapeutic purposes, originated in China more than 2,000 years ago. The Chinese believe an essential life energy, called *chi,* flows through the body along invisible channels, or meridians. There are thought to be at least 14 meridians connecting our organs with other parts of the body. Acupuncture and acupressure points lie on those meridians. When the flow of chi is blocked or out of balance, illness or pain results. Stimulation of specific points along the meridians can correct the flow of chi and block pain or restore health, according to the Chinese theory.

Although Western medicine has found no anatomical basis for the existence of acupuncture points or meridians, physicians have gradually come to accept the ability of acupuncture to relieve pain. According to the NIH consensus statement on acupuncture, these traditional Chinese medical concepts "are difficult to reconcile with contemporary biomedical information but continue to play an important role in the evaluation of patients and the formulation of treatment in acupuncture."[4]

The National Center for Complementary and Alternative Medicine takes a more pragmatic approach, stating, "Research has shown that acupuncture reduces nausea and vomiting after surgery and chemotherapy. It can also relieve pain. Researchers don't fully understand how acupuncture works. It might aid the activity of your body's pain-killing chemicals. It also might affect how you release chemicals that regulate blood pressure and flow."[5] Western scientists' best guess is that the meridians correspond to areas called trigger points that are rich in nerve endings. They believe stimulating these pressure points with needles produces a cascade of chemicals in the muscles, spinal cord, and brain that releases endorphins, the body's natural pain-killing substances.

A 2004 scientific study published in *Annals of Internal Medicine* found that acupuncture relieves knee arthritis symptoms, although the relief is often temporary and treatments must be repeated.[6] For best results, choose a therapist who is licensed and/or a graduate of a respected school of acupuncture and someone who is willing to work with your physician. About 10,000 acupuncturists currently practice in the U.S.; most are regulated by the state in which they reside. About 4,000 physicians have completed a recognized acupuncture training program.

Acupressure is somewhat less invasive than the acupuncture treatment modality, but it is believed to be much older. It relies on applying pressure with the hands and fingertips, and sometimes the feet, to the same points along the meridians used by acupuncturists to stimulate the body's natural self-healing capacities. When these points are pressed, they release muscle tension and promote the circulation of blood and the body's life force to aid in curing a range of muscle- and tendon-related ailments and injuries, as well as emotional ailments that may accompany chronic pain. Acupressure has the added advantage of being a modality that you can practice on yourself once properly instructed.

AQUA THERAPY

Also known as aquatic or pool therapy, aqua therapy amounts to an exercise program performed in the water. It uses the physical buoyancy of water to help healing by reducing joint stress. I have found this form of therapy to be of tremendous value for my patients with significant knee, hip or back arthritis, especially if they are overweight or obese. Buoyancy helps support their weight, reducing the force of stress on the joints. Decreasing the amount of joint stress makes it easier and less painful to exercise. At the same time, the viscous nature of water also provides more resistance, allowing patients to strengthen their muscles without using weights. The combination of resistance and buoyancy helps strengthen muscle groups with a lower level of joint stress than patients might experience on land. If you use a heated pool, the warmth of the water adds another level of therapeutic care that helps relax muscles and dilate blood vessels, increasing blood flow to injured areas. This aspect is especially helpful for anyone experiencing muscle spasms, back pain, or fibromyalgia syndrome. As always, check with your physician before using aqua therapy, especially if you have any form of cardiac disease.

SUMMING UP

Of the common alternatives to conventional medical care for arthritis and MSK pain, only massage therapy and acupuncture have so far been proven effective in clinical trials. While there is less rigorous medical evidence for the value of osteopathic and chiropractic care, many of my patients have been helped by both. Based on my personal experience, I have determined that acupuncture works well for knee, wrist-hand, and foot-ankle arthritis. Although a recent study appears to prove that acupuncture is effective in treating knee arthritis, clinical studies have shown conflicting results for acupuncture in chronic low-back pain.[7]

I have seen physical therapy be of tremendous value to those with chronic low-back pain, knee pain, and shoulder and elbow pain, as well as neck pain. For hip, lower-back, and neck pain, I have seen excellent results with osteopathy. Chiropractic treatments work well for lower-back arthritis, and therapeutic massage is effective for arthritis of the neck, lower back, and hip. I recommend acupuncture with very good results overall for chronic knee pain and neck pain.

And I have anecdotal evidence that aqua therapy works well for people with knee pain. One of my relatives, who is 65, is an electrical engineer and has suffered for years from knee arthritis that was caused by a cricket injury he sustained in his 20s. About seven years ago, I convinced him to start aqua therapy, and he now does it five days a week. He does not follow any of the other aspects of my Stop Pain Regimen, yet he claims that this one simple activity has kept up his mobility and minimized his pain despite a significantly arthritic knee.

Websites for Some Leading Organizations
of Integrative Medicine

American Physical Therapy Association	**apta.org**
American Osteopathy Association	**osteopathic.org**
American Massage Therapy Association	**amta.org**
American Association of Oriental Medicine (acupuncture)	**aaom.org**
American Chiropractic Association	**amerchiro.org**
American College of Rheumatology	**rheumatology.org**
American Academy of Physical Medicine and Rehabilitation	**aapmr.org**
American Association of Orthopaedic Surgeons	**aaos.org**

Chapter Eleven

The Mind-Body Connection and the Stress Factor

After the events of September 11, 2001, I saw a large spike in my practice of patients with new onset low back pain. I attributed this to the sudden rise in stress. While a small minority had no structural issues and their pain was mostly "in the mind," the vast majority suffered from a bulging of a spinal disc with resultant pain. Similarly large numbers of those with pre-existing chronic back pain that had been well managed experienced a sudden increase in pain after 9/11.

This is a powerful example of the impact that the mind has on the body, where a sudden increase in psychological stress can either contribute to the bulging of a disc or exacerbate an underlying chronic pain condition. For the vast majority with structural issues, the treatments I recommended consisted of standard care with incorporation of simple activities, such as walking or deep breathing to reduce the negative impacts of the stress. It was the small minority with no structural issues who needed psychological intervention, including the occasional use of antidepressant medications. Our understanding of the interrelationship of mind and body continues to grow, but we have a long way to travel. In my opinion, no treatment for chronic pain is complete without taking into account the powerful mind-body connection.

The interconnectedness of all levels of being has been a truism of the so-called New Age since at least the 1960s. According to this worldview, body, mind, and spirit (or soul) are intimately related and can affect each other profoundly on many different levels. The implications of the linkage between mind and body have become familiar today through many sources, including pioneering physicians and authors, notably Deepak Chopra, Bernie Siegel, Christiane Northrop, Caroline Myss, and others. But the seeds were planted much earlier in a couple of influential books that still have resonance today: *Anatomy of an Illness as Perceived by the Patient* by Norman Cousins, and *The Relaxation Response* by Dr. Herbert Benson. During the 1970s, these two books, while building on previous discoveries, revolutionized our understanding of the ability of the mind to influence the state of our physical health.

In some ways, *Anatomy of an Illness* was the more surprising of the two because its author was not a physician, yet his book has been cited as a milestone in the dawning awareness of our ability to tap into the body's powers to heal itself. Cousins (1915–1990) was a prominent political journalist, author, and world peace advocate, as well as an adjunct professor of medical humanities for the school of medicine at the University of California. Influenced by the groundbreaking work of endocrinologist Hans Selye, he had carried out research on the biochemistry of human emotions, which he long believed were the key to human beings' success in fighting illness. Late in life, Cousins was diagnosed with an especially debilitating form of arthritis now called ankylosing spondylitis, a degenerative disease that causes the breakdown of collagen, the fibrous tissue that binds together the body's cells. Almost completely paralyzed, Cousins was told that he had little chance of surviving. Instead of giving up, he prevailed on one of his doctors to help him implement his own healing program. He checked out of the hospital and into a hotel room, on the theory that overreliance on medication and routines that disrupted his sleep made the hospital "no place for a person who is seriously ill."

Ever the journalist, Cousins researched his condition and determined that the medication he was being given was depleting his body of Vitamin C, so with his doctor's help he began taking intravenous megadoses of the vitamin. Finally, based on his belief in the value of positive emotions, Cousins procured a movie projector and copies of comedy films, including several Marx Brothers movies and tapes of the popular TV program *Candid Camera*. "I made the joyous discovery that ten minutes of genuine belly laughter had an anesthetic effect and would give me at least two hours of pain-free sleep," Cousins wrote of the effects of watching comedy. "When the pain-killing effect of the laughter wore off, we would switch on the motion-picture projector again and, not infrequently, it would lead to another pain-free interval."

Although Cousins was definitely a pioneer, it's important to keep in mind that he did not reject Western medicine and science outright. He healed himself while working in close collaboration with a sympathetic doctor to overcome a supposedly irreversible disease. Studies related to Cousins's discovery have since shown that anger, depression, and pessimism weaken the immune response, as Dr. Selye had discovered decades earlier. These negative emotions also increase the time needed to recover from surgery and heal wounds, and probably contribute to higher death rates—just as we now know that being married or in a loving relationship definitely tends to extend life expectancy.

Before Cousins's book appeared, Dr. Herbert Benson, a cardiologist at Harvard Medical School, began to study the medical benefits of relaxation, and conclusively proved that simple relaxation techniques could lower blood pressure, slow the heart rate, and calm brain waves. In *The Relaxation Response*, published in 1975, he taught readers how to trigger this response by following a few simple instructions. In one sense, this was nothing new. More than 3,000 years ago, the yogis of India learned how to relax the mind and body through meditation and yoga, and left detailed accounts of their efforts in sacred scriptures from the *Rig Veda* to the *Yoga Sutras* of Patanjali. Stories had reached the West early in the 20th century of adepts in the Himalayas and Tibet who were able to slow their heartbeat and respiration virtually to a halt or raise their body temperature enough to dry sheets dipped in ice-cold water and wrapped around them in a cold environment. But because these powers of mind over matter were performed by ascetics with years of arduous practice behind them, they seemed out of reach for the average person.

Western medicine didn't start taking seriously the mind's ability to control the body until the 1920s, when Dr. Edmund Jacobson of the University of Chicago developed a technique he called "progressive relaxation," teaching patients to relax their muscles in sequence. Some years later Dr. Benson was approached by practitioners of Transcendental Meditation, a version of traditional Indian meditation promulgated by Maharishi Mahesh Yogi and popularized through Maharishi's encounter with the Beatles in the 1960s. Maharishi's adherents told Dr. Benson that they could control their blood pressure by entering into a meditative state and offered to prove it. Dr. Benson agreed to study them, but only if they would allow him to publish whatever he found, pro or con.

From his studies, Dr. Benson discovered that the meditators were indeed able to lower their blood pressure by meditating. At the time, most physicians still believed that the cardiovascular system was completely autonomic and could not be consciously controlled, so this appeared to be a significant breakthrough. Benson determined, moreover, that the ability to control blood pressure seemed to depend only on certain aspects of the meditative process and did not require a set of spiritual beliefs or even a specific Sanskrit mantra to work. He termed this basic principle the "relaxation response," and later defined it as an invaluable parallel to the "fight-or-flight" response, which had been discovered 60 years earlier. Dr. Benson considered the relaxation response to be "a second, equally essential survival mechanism—the ability to heal and rejuvenate our bodies."

RELAXATION FOR STRESS REDUCTION

Dr. Benson distilled the essential elements of the process of meditation as a physiological antidote to the stress of daily life, later modifying them in subsequent books, such as *Timeless Healing*. To be clear, this is quite distinct from traditional systems of meditation that have come down to us from the world's spiritual traditions, both Eastern and Western. If you are interested in meditation as a spiritual experience, you can explore the many formats that are available online, in books and at meditation centers. But for basic stress reduction as a way to alleviate pain, all you need to do is what Dr. Benson did: adapt the basics of meditation practice to a nonsectarian format for relaxation. I should mention that not all traditional meditation makes use of mantras, or repeated words. Some do, of course, and Eastern-based systems use mantras in Sanskrit, Japanese or other languages, while in the West, English mantras work quite well. Here is the essence of the relaxation response for stress reduction:

1. Pick a focus word or short phrase, such as "one," "peace," "love," "yes," or any mellifluous sound with no special associations. You can also use a religious word of significance to you.

2. Sit quietly in a comfortable position and close your eyes.

3. Uncross your legs and arms, place your feet flat on the floor.

4. Relax your muscles progressively from your feet to your face.

5. Breathe slowly and naturally through your nose, repeating your focus word silently as you exhale.

6. Assume a passive attitude, and don't be concerned with how well you're doing. When other thoughts come to mind, let them pass without judgment, and gently return to the repetition.

7. Do this for 10 to 20 minutes.

8. Continue sitting quietly for a minute or so before getting up, allowing other thoughts to return. Then open your eyes and sit for another minute before rising.

9. Practice this technique once or twice daily but at least an hour or two after eating a meal.

The key, according to Dr. Benson, is "to use a relaxation technique that will break the train of everyday thought, and decrease the activity of the sympathetic nervous system." That's the part of us that is responsible for the fight-or-flight response, among other things. The results of this simple technique have been impressive, and have been shown through many scientific studies to strengthen the immune system and produce a host of other medically valuable physiological changes. By lowering blood pressure and cholesterol levels, the research shows, relaxation may help make people less susceptible to viruses.[1]

Most significantly from my perspective, 75 percent of patients taking this program for sleep-onset insomnia (the inability to fall asleep, rather than to stay asleep) were cured and became normal sleepers, while the other 25 percent also improved, and most participants took significantly fewer sleep medications. Patients who suffered from anxiety, or mild to moderate depression were less anxious, depressed, angry, and hostile after using the stress-reduction techniques.[2]

I cannot emphasize enough the role of stress in creating pain and the importance of reducing stress to manage pain. The body is designed to handle the occasional stress response to danger, but prolonged levels of stress, along with the cortisol it releases into the bloodstream, have been shown to impair cognitive ability, thyroid function, and immune response. The effects of stress can also cause blood sugar imbalances, decrease bone density and muscle tissue, raise blood pressure, and increase abdominal fat, which is associated with heart disease and stroke. That's why it's so important to find ways to activate the body's inherent relaxation response to counteract the continual release of cortisol caused by chronic stress. Among the best and most often used methods of reducing stress are visualization or guided imagery, journaling, self-hypnosis, yoga, exercise, deep breathing, meditation, and even sex.

In the wake of Dr. Benson's discoveries, a number of other practitioners of meditation have helped spread the practice as a form of stress reduction, while taking nothing away from its potential spiritual value. Jon Kabat-Zinn, Ph.D., emeritus professor of medicine at the University of Massachusetts and the author of several influential books including *Full Catastrophe Living*, has developed Mindfulness-Based Stress Reduction, a popular short-term therapeutic system that combines elements of meditation and yoga. Kabat-Zinn is largely responsible for the adoption of meditation by hospitals and health-care practitioners. Today, practices like Kabat-Zinn's continue to be used and expanded by knowledgeable physicians and therapists in a surprising variety of ways. Many of them are fairly simple and require no special training to make use of.

DEEP BREATHING

One of the best and easiest ways I know of to reduce pain is proper breathing, by which I mean slow, deep breathing. In the course of a single day, we take somewhere in the neighborhood of 21,000 breaths. Most of us breathe like rabbits, taking short, shallow breaths all day long. Those shallow breaths activate the receptors in the upper lobes of the lungs and stimulate the sympathetic nervous system. Those receptors are designed to trigger responses that are beneficial during emergencies, speeding up blood flow and releasing adrenalin. But it's deleterious to your health to activate those stress receptors regularly. When you breathe deeply as I will instruct you below, you stimulate the lower lobes of the lungs and activate the parasympathetic nervous system. This has a calming effect on both body and mind, and helps reduce pain measurably.

More parasympathetic activity means less stress and, so, better heart health.

Natural, or diaphragmatic, breathing is the way nature intended us to breathe—through the nose. Sit on a chair with both feet flat on the floor. You should be comfortable—not slumped back in the chair but more toward the front, with your spine straight and your chin slightly tucked to keep the back of your neck properly aligned. Loosen your clothing so that you can breathe comfortably.

1. Place one palm on your navel, the other on the small of your back.

2. Breathe deeply through your nose. Breathe only through your nose, as this purifies, warms, and moistens the air as it enters the breathing passage.

3. Consciously expand the belly and small of the back on the inhalation, and push out the air during the exhalation. You should be able to feel your abdomen and, to a lesser extent, the small of your back expand slightly on inhalation and contract with exhalation.

4. As the abdomen expands and you continue breathing, you can direct excess air up into the chest cavity, expanding the diaphragm—a muscle that extends across the base of the rib cage.

5. For a basic cycle, inhale to a count of four and hold for a count of six. Then exhale to a count of six and hold for a count of four before repeating the cycle.

6. Repeat this cycle for at least three minutes, and preferably for five to ten minutes at a sitting.

VISUALIZATION

One way to make things happen is to visualize them. Although the practice of visualization began with spiritual adepts, it has been recognized as so effective that athletes and coaches use it regularly to enhance physical performance. But you can also use visualization to enhance states of psychological calm and tranquility and to relieve pain. As I have discussed frequently throughout this book, chronic pain has a psychological component that can make it even harder to manage. But we can use psychological techniques to counter pain as well. You can begin teaching yourself visualization by combining it with the breathing practice I've just shown you. Once you've done the breathing routine a few times, you should be ready to add some visualization elements to it. Begin this way:

1. As you breathe in through your nose with your eyes closed, visualize a ray of white light coming in through the crown of your head, and traveling down through your throat, heart, and navel to the base of your spine.

2. Hold the light there for a moment before exhaling.

3. As you exhale, visualize the light turning to a smoky, dark gray color with a thick texture.

4. Now see the smoke dissipating from the base of your spine down into the earth.

5. When you have finished exhaling, hold for a moment until you begin to inhale a new ray of bright white light entering the crown of your head and flowing down your spinal column to the base of the spine.

6. Once more, hold the light there for a moment before exhaling a column of dark gray smoke down into the earth.

Imagine that the white or gold light you are inhaling consists of healing energy, and the dark smoke you exhale is your pain, which you send out of your body and deep into the ground. With each exhalation, allow the dark, almost black smoke to become a little lighter. Continue the visualization until the smoke becomes light gray and finally white.

You can devise many variations on this method of visualization, either by yourself or in collaboration with a trained professional. Bornali Basu, Ph.D., who clinically supervises trainees at NYU Medical School and Columbia Teacher's College in New York, combines the techniques of deep breathing, relaxation, and visualization in her practice, gearing particular programs to each individual client. Basu herself suffers from migraines, and has developed a series of visualizations to help diminish their severity: "I live in the city, so I like to imagine an apartment building lit up on one side and all dark on the other side. As you breathe out, visualize one light going out at a time. As each light shuts off, allow some of the pain to diminish."

The first step is to accept the presence of pain, but then to look for details that may be clues to alleviating its hold on you. "Your pain is real," Basu says. "We're not here to debate that, but to give you a little more control over your experience." At certain times of day, for instance, the pain may be more or less intense. When we think about stressful things, we probably feel the pain more severely. By addressing questions like when the pain occurs and the severity of the occurrence, we can see a gradation in the level of pain, and then link that gradation to what is going on at any given moment. People who have suffered pain for a long time may believe they will always have pain. But that is merely a preconception that amounts to a false belief system. Through breathing and visualization, you can counter such belief systems and loosen their grip.

DEPRESSION AND PAIN

Pain and depression are closely related, especially when we consider the effects of chronic pain. Pain can cause depression; depression can cause pain and increased pain sensitivity. Indeed, a recent report from the Harvard Medical School says, "People with chronic pain have three times the average risk of developing psychiatric symptoms—usually mood or anxiety disorders—and depressed patients have three times the average risk of developing chronic pain."[3] Think about that for a moment. Most people who suffer from chronic pain and depression fail to make the connection. They may say they have been depressed for a long time and the pain is a recent phenomenon, or vice versa. But rest assured that a direct link usually exists between pain and depression, and that one often begins not so long after the other has taken hold.

Acute pain that lasts a short time may make you feel sad or even angry, but chronic pain that goes on and on with no hope of respite can be downright depressing. This connection also runs the other way, though. According to Dr. Daniel K. Hall-Flavin, a psychiatrist with the Mayo Clinic, "Sometimes, depression causes unexplained physical symptoms—such as back pain or headaches. In other cases, depression may increase your response to pain, or at least increase the suffering associated with pain." He adds, "Sometimes pain and depression create a vicious cycle."[4] Part of the reason for that cycle may be that pain and depression share common pathways in the emotional region of the brain, according to some recent research, and the same chemical messengers that control pain also control mood. This appears to explain why antidepressant medications also have central pain-blocking properties and have been used frequently for pain.

In my experience, chronic pain can sometimes create so much anxiety and grief that I often recommend, along with following my recommendations for diet, exercise, and medication, that my patients who have an anxiety or depression component see a psychotherapist or, if there is need, a psychiatrist. As I noted in my discussion of fibromyalgia syndrome, its symptoms include apparently inexplicable muscle pain and tenderness at certain "trigger points" on the body (see illustration, p. 37), despite an absence of observable nerve damage. People with FMS often show highly active pain centers during brain scans, and the disorder is closely associated with depression. One theory holds that some kind of brain malfunction may heighten sensitivity to both pain and mood changes. "Depression leads to isolation and isolation leads to further depression," according to the Harvard Medical School report cited above. "Pain causes fear of movement, and immobility creates the conditions for further pain. When depression is treated, pain often fades into the background, and when pain goes away, so does much of the suffering that causes depression."[5]

A 1992 study showed that major depression, or clinical depression, is four times greater in people with chronic back pain than in the general population.[6] And yet the whole issue of whether pain causes depression or depression causes pain is controversial, writes Dr. Michael Clark of the Department of Psychiatry and Behavioral Sciences at Johns Hopkins University School of Medicine. "Many of the criteria traditionally used to diagnose major depression overlap with the symptoms experienced by patients with chronic pain."[7] But that has also opened the door to the use of antidepressants to treat both pain and depression. Because, as noted, pain and depression share the same pathways in the brain, some medications work for both, as we will see in some detail in the following chapter on prescription pain medications. In my experience, the connection is pretty clear.

About one year ago I saw a 47-year-old woman named Jackie who was going through a divorce and had recently lost her father. She complained that she had suffered from low-back pain for six months. While I was taking her history, it became clear to me that her pain was neither exacerbated nor alleviated by walking or sitting or standing for a long time. Most chronic low-back pain caused by a physical problem in the spine is made better or worse by certain activities, but on exam, no movements exacerbated her pain. Her back pain was severe and had begun a month after her father passed away. I determined that the pain she was feeling was not actually from a physical condition but instead was a result of the mental stress and anguish she was feeling.

I asked Jackie to see one of my colleagues who is a psychiatrist, as well as a psychotherapist who specializes in chronic pain. After she started on an antidepressant medication and had a few sessions with the psychotherapist, her pain went down remarkably. I also asked her to walk daily for 20 to 30 minutes and ice her back, because I thought these were possible placebo treatments that might act synergistically with the psychotherapy and antidepressants for therapeutic effects. Within six weeks, Jackie's pain was gone entirely. As I've said, the percentage of people who have significant pain without any structural abnormalities is low. The vast majority of chronic pain sufferers usually have some structural problem, along with underlying anxiety or depression that might make the pain worse. For these people, mind-body therapies remain a valuable low-tech treatment to manage the pain.

PART IV

CONVENTIONAL MEDICAL OPTIONS

Chapter Twelve

Prescription Medications, Invasive Procedures, and Surgical Options

You may wonder why, if I have such reservations about prescription medications for pain relief, I include them in the book at all. I believe in the old saying of Sir Francis Bacon, "Knowledge is power." If your physician prescribes the drugs in this chapter but fails to warn you of the side effects, or if you see commercials on TV that make them sound like panaceas, at least you'll be forewarned. Keep my book handy and refer to it before taking any prescription or OTC pain meds. By the same token, if other pain-relief options I've recommended aren't working for you, then you can resort to these medications armed with the knowledge that they work best when used for short durations.

So, although I firmly believe that you can relieve most chronic pain without taking prescription medications, including painkillers, I'm also enough of a realist to base my recommendations on my direct experiences with patients. For a certain percentage of people in pain, the safest approaches don't yield results. I'm always sensitive to their pain, so I try not to be doctrinaire about the treatment options I offer. I do remind my patients, however, of the potential downside of these options and tell them to think of these treatments as stopgap interventions rather than continuing courses of treatment. If someone is in excruciating pain, so intense that he can barely walk and can't sleep at night, he may need an injection or prescription painkillers. But once the crisis has passed and the patient is able to function without pain, I introduce other options.

PRESCRIPTION NSAIDS

Even when intervening with conventional treatments, I begin with the safest and proceed further up the risk ladder only if less risky treatments don't produce the desired pain relief. The safest conventional option is the use of prescription NSAIDs, in pill, patch, or topical form. All NSAIDs, including the lone COX-2 still on the market, are associated with higher risk of heart disease and stroke, especially if you take them for a long period of time or have a history of high blood pressure or diabetes. In the short run, however, especially if you don't have any of the risk factors just mentioned, they can reduce both pain and inflammation. But just remember, all NSAIDs, both oral and topical, treat the symptoms of pain but do not address the cause.

Each NSAID has specific advantages and disadvantages, and it helps to choose the one that best suits your situation. I'm afraid it's a little like choosing investments; the vehicles that offer the biggest return on your money also carry the largest risk. Sometimes you're better off investing in a bank CD than playing the market. But if you do make high-risk investments, it's better to do so in the short term, and the same is true of using any medication that has a risk attached that grows greater the longer you stay with it.

Some of the most commonly used NSAIDs, along with their associated advantages and disadvantages, are listed in the chart on the next page.

As I explained in the discussion of OTC NSAIDs in Chapter Eight, these drugs work by interfering with the Cox-1 and Cox-2 production of prostaglandins and lead to ulcers and bleeding in the stomach and intestine. (Prostaglandins are hormone-like substances that help support many physiological functions.)

MOST COMMON NSAIDS		
Drug	**Advantage**	**Disadvantage**
Arthrotec	Most potent	High side effects, should not be taken by people with cardiac arrhythmias
Lodine	Moderate potency	Moderate stomach irritation
Naprosyn, ibuprofen (prescription strength)	Moderate potency	Moderate stomach irritation
Mobic, Relafen	Mild potency	Very mild side effects
Voltaren XR	High potency	Moderate stomach irritation
Celebrex	Low risk of ulcers	Expensive, mild potency, risk of heart disease

The same warnings that were given for the use of OTC NSAIDs apply to prescription NSAIDs. Patients who take other medications, such as blood-thinning drugs, other NSAIDs, oral steroids, lithium, or methotrexate should alert their doctor when starting any prescription to avoid dangerous drug interactions. Remember that prolonged use of NSAIDs can result in higher blood pressure and can also cause kidney problems, especially in patients with diabetes. To avoid these complications during long-term use, I recommend "drug holidays" along with blood tests to measure kidney function. Patients with diabetes should have these blood tests twice a year. Patients at risk for heart disease should have an annual blood test. In general, however, it is best to avoid long-term use of NSAIDs altogether and only take them in times of acute pain.

Topical NSAID applications (ointment, gel, skin patches) are all subject to the same warnings as their oral counterparts, thus the same cautions need to be taken when using multiple medications and when determining the length of time you can safely use them. Newer types of prescription topical analgesics that contain NSAIDs, such as diclofenac (Voltaren, Emulgel), help reduce the swelling and inflammation of soft tissues (tendons, ligaments, muscles) caused by trauma or osteoarthritis and rheumatoid arthritis, and so decrease pain. The main limitation of these topicals is their inability to get a sufficient amount of active ingredients to the pain-causing area. The Flector Topical Patch (diclofenac epolamine) is an NSAID for the treatment of acute pain due to minor injuries, but it is also used to treat chronic conditions including fibromyalgia and arthritis.

COX-2 INHIBITORS

Because so many people expose themselves to risk by taking NSAIDs, scientists developed a new class of drugs in the 1990s to decrease the chances of ulcers, bleeding, and perforation of the stomach or intestine. While COX-2 inhibitors are actually a type of NSAID, I'm setting them apart because their pain-relief mechanism works differently. As I mentioned before, NSAIDs block both Cox-1 and Cox-2. While they both produce prostaglandins, Cox-2 produces the prostaglandins that trigger inflammation, while Cox-1 (the "good" Cox) produces the prostaglandins that enable the stomach to protect itself against bleeding. The new class of drugs became known as Cox-2 inhibitors, because they do not inhibit Cox-1, and so reduce pain while significantly diminishing the risk of digestive side effects including bleeding ulcers. But as often happens with new pharmaceutical drugs, the Cox-2 inhibitors were soon causing more harm than good, and all but Celebrex were withdrawn from the market by the manufacturers because of an increased chance of heart attack. The manufacturers of Celebrex (celecoxib) claim that there is no greater risk of heart attacks from their drug than from other NSAIDs; however, all prescription NSAIDs, including celecoxib, carry the FDA's sternest warning, stating that they may increase the chance of heart attack or stroke, which can lead to death.

Studies conducted by independent researchers without the financial sponsorship of the drug companies have not been completed, and until results from independent analyses such as these become available, the use of celecoxib should be carefully considered. Celecoxib not only increases blood pressure, but also can increase the risk of blood clot formation, putting patients at greater risk for heart disease. For these reasons, the use of celecoxib should be limited to people who have low risk of heart disease and high blood pressure and cannot take NSAIDs because they have ulcers.

I recommend that those who use celecoxib take a baby aspirin every day to minimize the risk of heart disease (small-dose aspirin and COX-2 inhibitors don't interfere with each other), and that they take celecoxib only in spurts. If patients must use it for six months or more, I advise them to take a drug holiday one day a week, as with NSAIDs. Individuals with diabetes should have a blood test twice a year to measure the effect of the drug on their kidneys. Other patients should have the blood test once a year. People with arthritis and rheumatoid arthritis may also use celecoxib if everything else has failed and they still have pain. If the patient has a history of gastrointestinal problems, a proton pump inhibitor, which is a class of drugs that reduce the production of gastric acid, may be needed to protect the stomach. Because of the controversy over the role of COX-2 drugs in increasing risk for heart attack, physicians are prescribing celecoxib less often as the initial drug to control pain. As in the past, the physician and the patient in partnership have to make practical and cost-benefit decisions when a patient is in constant pain. For all these reasons, I refer you back to my discussion of safer herbal remedies to reduce inflammation and pain in Chapter Seven.

Unless we solve the problem of blood clotting and heart disease as a result of COX-2 use, the future of these drugs remains questionable. And it bears repeating that all oral medications, whether OTC or prescription, carry risks with repeated use.

ANTIDEPRESSANTS

As noted in the preceding chapter, pain and depression are often linked in one way or another. But depression itself has many other causes. Sadness at the loss of a loved one or over a divorce is normal, but these losses can also trigger a more profound depressive episode. Almost any major life change can do the same, including job promotions or layoffs, moving to a new area, or learning that you have a potentially dangerous medical condition. In recent years, scientists and researchers have come to the conclusion that clinical depression—as distinguished from occasional feelings of sadness or discouragement—can be the result of several factors working together. Although researchers are not entirely certain, the three most important causes seem to be biological, genetic, and environmental factors.

Environmental factors, like the divorce or job loss mentioned above, can be the trigger for depression, while the other two factors are closely related to each other. Genetic predisposition may be the result of faulty brain chemistry, caused by fluctuations in the levels of certain brain chemicals essential to healthy functioning, especially serotonin, dopamine, and norepinephrine (nor-ep-ih-NEF-rin). Scientists believe a deficiency in serotonin may cause the sleep problems, irritability, and anxiety associated with depression. Low levels of dopamine reduce the ability to feel pleasure and enthusiasm. Insufficient levels of norepinephrine, which regulates alertness and arousal, may lead to the systemic fatigue and dejected mood that many with depression feel. All three chemicals are known as neurotransmitters, made by the nerve cells in the brain that send messages back and forth between the cells. MRIs and brain tissue samples of depressed patients have shown that these neurotransmitters are below normal levels.

The chemistry may be complicated, but researchers have found ways to restore low levels of these vital neurotransmitters using various kinds of drugs known collectively as antidepressants. And many physicians have found a so-called off-label use—the use of a prescription medication to treat a condition other than what it was designed for—for antidepressants in the treatment of certain chronic pain conditions. However, their use as pain relievers is now so commonplace as to make that designation unnecessary. Antidepressants are among the more effective and commonly used medications for chronic pain.

The oldest class of antidepressants is called tricyclics. Developed in the 1950s, they worked to inhibit the reabsorption (reuptake) of serotonin and norepinephrine, and, to a lesser extent, dopamine, by brain cells. They also block other cell receptors, which accounts for many of their side effects, the most notable of which are weight gain, drowsiness, and dry mouth. The tricyclics are named after the drugs' molecular structure, which contains three rings of atoms, and include a number of generics that have long been in use and are considered relatively safe. The one most frequently used for pain, especially low-back pain, is amitriptyline (Elavil), although several others have been used with some success, including (with most common brand names in parentheses) imipramine (Tofranil), clomipramine (Anafranil), nortriptyline (Pamelor), desipramine (Norpramin), and doxepin (Sinequan).

The tricyclics were eventually supplanted by a newer group of antidepressants called SSRIs. The acronym stands for selective serotonin reuptake inhibitors; the first and best known was fluoxetine (Prozac), which came on the U.S. market in 1987. SSRIs get their name from the process of keeping more serotonin available in the brain, which enhances the sending of nerve impulses and somehow improves one's mood—although, once again, scientists aren't sure exactly how this works. SSRIs are called "selective" because they seem to affect only serotonin, not the other major neurotransmitters involved with mood. For whatever reason, the SSRIs have proven somewhat more effective, and their side effects are more easily tolerated, although these can include sexual dysfunction, both as reduced desire and difficulty achieving orgasm, as well as nausea, weight gain, and restlessness. In general, these effects haven't been as hard for most people to tolerate as those associated with tricyclics.

Another class of antidepressants, known as SNRIs (serotonin-norepinephron reuptake inhibitors), is believed to have better pain-relief properties than the SSRIs. SNRIs increase the levels of both serotonin and norepinephrine available in the brain, which has also made them popular antidepressants. Duloxetine (Cymbalta) has been approved for relieving the pain of fibromyalgia. But the high side effect profiles of SNRIs make them a less than optimal choice among antidepressants for treating pain.

Each group and each individual drug has specific advantages and drawbacks, which are summarized on the chart below. Tricyclics are used most often to treat the pain of nerve damage from diabetes and shingles (postherpetic neuralgia), as well as tension and migraine headaches, fibromyalgia, and low-back pain. The painkilling mechanism of these drugs is no better understood than their effect on depression, although they are believed to increase the presence of neurotransmitters in the spinal cord that reduce pain signals. Unfortunately, they tend not to work immediately. You may have to take a tricyclic antidepressant for several weeks before it starts reducing your pain—just as when you take them to relieve depression. That drawback may be counterbalanced by the fact that their few side effects (including drowsiness, dry mouth, constipation, weight gain, difficulty with urination, and changes in blood pressure) are usually mild, because the dosages that are effective for pain are typically lower than those used for depression. The best way to reduce or prevent side effects is to start at a low dose and slowly increase the amount, as you would do when treating depression. In general, SSRIs are a better bet than tricyclics for pain relief, as they have fewer side effects, especially regarding weight gain.

ANTIDEPRESSANTS FOR PAIN RELIEF			
Brand (Generic)	**Class**	**Benefits**	**Drawbacks**
Elavil (amitriptyline)	Tricyclic	Good pain relief	Weight gain, dry mouth, drowsiness
Pamelor (nortriptyline)	Tricyclic	Very good pain relief, especially for chronic back pain	Same as Elavil
Lexapro (escitalopram)	SSRI	Excellent for pain relief	Moderate side effects

Prozac (fluoxetine) Paxil (paroxetine) Celexa (citalopram) Zoloft (sertraline)	SSRI	Generally good for pain relief	Moderate side effects
Wellbutrin (bupropion)	SSRI	Good for pain and anxiety	Moderate side effects
Cymbalta (duloxetine)	SNRI	Good pain relief	High side effect profile
Effexor (venlafaxine)	SNRI	Above average pain relief	High side effect profile

NERVE MEMBRANE STABILIZERS

A class of drugs originally designed to treat seizures of various types has also been used to alleviate certain nerve-related pain. Nerve membrane stabilizers diminish pain caused by damaged nerves and maintain a feeling of balance and well-being. Without going too far into the complex way they work, I will note that these drugs seek to maximize the presence of GABA (gamma-aminobutyric acid), a neurotransmitter that regulates brain and nerve cell activity by inhibiting the number of neurons firing in the brain. Sometimes referred to as the brain's natural calming agent, GABA induces relaxation, reduces stress and anxiety, and increases alertness. People with a GABA deficiency often experience anxiety symptoms, irritability, headaches, hypertension, palpitations, and seizures. Dr. Ray Sahelian, author of *Mind Boosters,* writes, "GABA is the most important and widespread inhibitory neurotransmitter in the brain. Excitation in the brain must be balanced with inhibition. Too much excitation can lead to restlessness, irritability, insomnia, and even seizures. GABA is able to induce relaxation, analgesia, and sleep."[1]

Different medications use different means to stimulate GABA production and maintain levels of GABA, just as antidepressants seek to maximize levels of the neurotransmitter serotonin in the brain. GABA also helps produce endorphins, the brain chemicals that create a feeling of well-being. These generic drugs include (with brand names in parentheses) pregabalin (Lyrica), gabapentin (Neurontin), tiagabine (Gabitril), topiramate (Topamax), carbamazepine (Tegretol), lamotrigine (Lamictyl)), phenytoin (Dilantin), valproate (Depakote), and clonazepam (Klonopin). You should know that although some of these drugs can be effective at increasing feelings of relaxation and calm, at the wrong dosage they may also make you feel sedated or sluggish. You'll need to work closely with your physician to decide which nerve stabilizers may be effective for you, and at what dosage. Lyrica is the only one in this class approved for fibromyalgia. The biggest drawback of this class continues to be the relatively high incidence of side effects, such as excessive drowsiness or balance and dizziness issues.

Transdermal patches containing lidocaine, a local anesthetic, marketed as Lidoderm, were developed to relieve the peripheral pain of shingles (herpes zoster). But early studies are suggesting that lidocaine patches may provide significant relief for low-back pain with few adverse side effects. Make sure you don't use Lidoderm patches for more than 12 hours per day in order to avoid lidocaine toxicity, which can have adverse effects.

ORAL STEROIDS

Oral steroids are a non-narcotic type of prescription medication with powerful anti-inflammatory properties. They can sometimes be an effective treatment for severe acute flare-ups of MSK pain, especially low-back issues with mostly leg pain or rheumatoid arthritis flare-ups. Because of the potentially hazardous side effects from long-term use, I prescribe them only for short periods of time, one to two weeks at most. In my opinion, they are very useful for flare-ups of autoimmune diseases like rheumatoid arthritis, but have limited efficacy for acute flare-ups of sciatica.

It's important to note that the steroids I'm discussing here are *catabolic* steroids, also called *corticosteroids*. They should not be confused with *anabolic* steroids, which result in the buildup of cellular tissue, especially in muscles. Anabolic steroids are used legitimately to treat chronic wasting conditions, such as cancer and AIDS. But because long-term use can result in severe liver and heart damage, their abuse by athletes and bodybuilders to gain a competitive advantage is now banned by most major professional sports organizations. Corticosteroids have the opposite effect of anabolics, as they break down muscle mass rather than building it up, but they have potent anti-inflammatory properties to reduce significant inflammation with resultant pain and swelling.

Oral steroids come in many forms, but are usually ordered as a Medrol Dose Pack; patients start with a high dose for initial pain relief and then taper down to a lower dose over five or six days. The pack contains methylprednisolone tablets, a glucocorticoid (corticosteroid) that helps to reduce swelling, redness, itching, and allergic reactions. It can be used to treat severe allergies, skin problems, asthma, arthritis, and other conditions, including multiple sclerosis. Generic Medrol Dose Pack tablets are also available.

Oral catabolic steroids should be used on a short-term basis, as a number of potential complications are associated with long-term usage, from weight gain and stomach ulcers to osteoporosis, collapse of the hip joint, and other complications. People with diabetes should be very careful with oral steroids, because the medication increases blood sugar. Steroids should not be used in the presence of active infections, such as in the sinuses or urinary tract.

NARCOTIC PAINKILLERS AND OPIOIDS

Early researchers into the mechanisms of pain and pain relief have observed that most analgesics derive from just a couple of natural plants and then from synthetic versions of each. We have seen that aspirin was created from chemicals found in the bark of the willow tree, and aspirin substitutes have been synthesized along the lines of those compounds. Likewise, morphine was derived from the opium poppy, and most opioids and synthetic opiates followed suit. Opioids are the most potent painkillers we know, but partly because of that they are subject to the greatest abuse, including addiction. All the opiates and their derivatives are habit-forming.

Propoxyphene (Darvon) is probably the mildest of the narcotic painkillers, used for mild to moderate pain with or without fever. Hydrocodone is a semi-synthetic opioid similar in its effects to morphine; it can lead to dependence, tolerance, and addiction when abused. (As I noted in the Introduction, hydrocodone is the most commonly prescribed medication *of any category* in the United States today, and I suspect the reason is patient demand!) Oxycodone is a more potent narcotic analgesic. A controlled-release version of oxycodone, sold under the brand name OxyContin, has much more serious side effects. Both drugs are prescribed for moderate to severe pain, but the potential for abuse is obvious. When OxyContin tablets are crushed to a fine powder and snorted or injected, the effect is somewhat like heroin, and can be life-threatening.

In July 2009, a federal advisory panel recommended to the Food and Drug Administration that it ban Percocet and Vicodin, two of the most popular prescription painkillers in the world, both of which combine a narcotic with acetaminophen, the ingredient found in popular OTC products like Tylenol and Excedrin. A half dozen other such prescription painkillers also contain acetaminophen, including Darvoset N-100, and it's possible that the FDA may consider banning all of them for the same reason. As patients develop a tolerance and increase their dosage of these painkillers, they are also increasing their intake of acetaminophen, often to dangerous levels that can result in liver damage. Most people are probably unaware that these painkillers contain acetaminophen, which generally appears on the pharmacy label as APAP, an abbreviation of its European name. If you are taking painkillers that also contain acetaminophen, make sure you limit the amount to less than 3,000 milligrams per day.

Tramadol hydrochloride (Ultram) and tramadol with acetaminophen (Ultracet) are central nervous system depressants used for treating moderate to severe pain. Studies show that patients are no more likely to abuse this drug than normal NSAIDs, and it is not regulated as a controlled substance by the Drug Enforcement Administration. And yet, although tramadol is not an opioid, some controversy exists regarding the liability of dependence or addiction. The prescribing information for Ultram warns that tramadol "may induce psychological and physical dependence of the morphine type," and some patients have reported uncontrollable withdrawal-like nervous tremors when weaned off the medication too quickly. For that reason it's best to use tramadol only for limited periods, and to monitor closely its discontinuation.

Although opioids have little risk of the health dangers of steroids and NSAIDs, apart from their potential for abuse, they do have side effects including dizziness, drowsiness, or headache; nervousness, tremor, or anxiety; nausea, vomiting, constipation, or diarrhea; and itching, dry mouth, or sweating.

Perhaps the most significant reason to avoid using opioids except in extreme cases is that they create what I consider a downward spiral effect. To begin, the potency of all opioids for pain relief tends to diminish over time. Your system becomes used to them, and you need increasingly larger doses to achieve the same analgesic effect. At the same time, as I note elsewhere in this book, opioids tend to inhibit REM sleep, and the more you take them, the less REM sleep you will experience. Yet sleep, especially deep sleep, and REM sleep in particular, is one of the most important elements in any pain-relief regimen. Your body needs serious downtime to refresh and renew itself and allow its own natural painkillers to go to work. So after a time, the paradoxical result of using opioids may be *more* pain and greater sensitivity to pain.

NARCOTIC DRUGS			
Generic (Brand)	Potency	Value	Dangers
Propoxyphene (Darvon)	Mild potency	Low effect on mental activity	Addiction potential
Hydrocodone (Vicodin)	Moderate potency	Low effect on mental activity	High addiction potential

Oxycodone (Percocet)	High potency	Potentially high impact on mental activity	High addiction potential
Oxycodone timed-release (OxyContin)	High potency	Longer-lasting pain relief; high impact on mental activity	Extremely addictive; life-threatening when crushed into powder and inhaled

I discussed the value of transdermal patches in Chapter Eight, and much the same goes for patches that deliver narcotic painkillers, with some very important caveats, or warnings. Like oral narcotics, skin patches conveying opioid drugs should be used only under extreme circumstances to relieve MSK pain, as they can be addictive and occasionally can result in death through overdose. Because the drug is absorbed through the skin into the bloodstream, these patches can relieve pain for up to three days from a single application. The benefit is that patients don't have to take multiple doses of oral medications to control pain. On the downside, the FDA is investigating deaths and overdoses that have occurred with both brand-name (Duragesic) and generic fentanyl patches. Fentanyl should be used only for long-term or chronic pain requiring continuous, around-the-clock narcotic pain relief that is not helped by other less powerful pain medicines or less-frequent dosing. Because fentanyl can be very addictive, I don't recommend it for most patients.

INVASIVE PROCEDURES AND SURGICAL OPTIONS

If everything I've suggested here fails to do the job, you always have the option of minimally invasive or surgical procedures. These options, however, should be your last resort. Any medical procedure or surgery carries with it the risk of complications that could lead to even more serious pain. Also, the chance of success varies based on your condition and the procedure you get. Those chances improve if you are in the subgroup of patients we like to refer to as "well selected." That simply means that you meet the criteria for a given procedure—for example, that you experience pain mainly in the leg, or the low back, say, and that you have had the pain for more than six months (chronic pain). You and your physician should be able to determine whether you fit the designation of "well selected" for any given procedure.

Patients suffering primarily from leg pain caused by a disc bulge are well selected for a transforaminal epidural, which is usually effective. A transforaminal is a special type of epidural injection that is delivered to precisely where the disc and the nerve meet to reduce inflammation and so the pain. These injections have been shown to reduce significant amounts of pain over the long term when combined with the proper exercise regimen, according to clinical trial data published by my colleagues and me in 2002. If the epidural doesn't relieve the pain, a surgical discectomy—removing part of the disc—can be very effective.

A total hip replacement is one of the most successful orthopedic surgical procedures we have; over 95 percent of patients with end-stage hip arthritis report excellent pain relief from this form of surgery.

The outcome for knee replacement, though, is not as good. Some 85 percent of patients report good pain relief, but 15 percent still complain of either residual pain or loss of motion. Knee and hip replacements usually last 15 to 20 years and then have to be redone.

Patients suffering from spinal stenosis with mostly leg pain find transforaminal epidurals are helpful when combined with proper exercises. A laminectomy (surgery to remove the portion of the vertebral bone called the lamina) can be effective at alleviating leg pain, but in the long run it may bring on more back pain, because one of the bones that supports the spine is cut away during the procedure, placing more stress on the joints in the spine.

For those suffering from mostly back pain without much leg pain because of tears in the disc, the success rates go down quite a bit. Their chances improve, however, with a nonsurgical procedure called intradiscal electrothermal therapy, or IDET, as it is known commercially. IDET is a new, minimally invasive technique that involves threading a flexible catheter into the disc under fluoroscopic guidance. The catheter heats the outer ring of the disc (recall my jelly donut metaphor), ultimately disabling the pain receptors. (Clinical studies suggest that IDET might be effective in, at most, two-thirds of well-selected patients with intractable low-back pain due to tears in the disc without any evidence of degeneration, but its efficacy hasn't been tested in randomized, controlled clinical trials.)

Other nonsurgical interventions for those with mostly back pain, such as spinal cord stimulators or intrathecal pumps have success rates of less than 50 percent. For the same group of patients, the success rates for spinal fusion—a highly invasive surgical procedure—are below 50 percent. (Fusion is surgery that seeks to correct spinal problems by fusing together two or more vertebrae, using bone grafts, metal rods and screws.) I ask this subgroup to avoid surgical interventions altogether.

Spinal stenosis patients with primarily back pain can try a minimally invasive procedure called radiofrequency denervation (RFD) if the majority of their pain comes from the facet joints of the spine. For well-selected patients in this group the success rate is 80 percent, but the procedure has to be repeated every year or two.

The success rates involving surgery for this group of stenosis patients with mostly back pain are again below 50 percent. If my patients don't get significant pain relief with radiofrequency, I urge them not to consider surgical intervention, because the success rate is so low. In my opinion, the only good candidates for fusion are those who have spinal stenosis with a bony slip called spondylolisthesis (SPON-dih-lo-liss-THEE-sis) and who experience most of their pain in the leg. Spondylolisthesis refers to the displacement of a vertebra or the vertebral column in relation to the vertebrae below. (This is sometimes referred to incorrectly as a "slipped disc," when it is really a slipped bone. Remember, the vertebrae are the bones; the discs are the jelly donuts between the bones. Isn't this fun?)

Regardless of how invasive a procedure you may require, the Stop Pain Regimen should remain your basic course of therapy for trying to live with less pain and less dependence on narcotics while enhancing the quality of your life. In short, have the procedure if you must, but also continue following the advice in this book regarding diet, exercise, and the use of dietary supplements.

This brings to a close just about everything you should know regarding MSK pain—what causes it, what makes it worse, and how to alleviate it. I may have skipped over a few procedures that are either extremely technical or of little practical use. Of course, there are always areas that don't come up in the logical course of explaining such a complex topic as pain, so I've reserved a small section at the end of the book for some of the most frequently asked questions that people pose to me regarding pain.

PART V

FREQUENTLY ASKED QUESTIONS

Chapter Thirteen

Everything You Wanted to Know about Pain

Every day I see patients who suffer from various forms of chronic pain. They come in with many misconceptions or a complete lack of knowledge about their symptoms—what's good, what's bad; what should they do in certain instances. While I've heard hundreds of specific questions, there are some that occur with a much greater frequency. The following is a list of the most frequently asked questions that I've heard throughout my years of treating chronic pain.

1. No pain, no gain. Myth or reality?

That saying was a favorite of aerobics instructors and personal trainers during the 1980s and '90s, but it embodies a concept that is totally erroneous. Pain is your body's way of telling you that something is wrong. Working through it can cause serious problems. When you start a new exercise regimen, a slight increase in discomfort, muscle aches, or fatigue is normal, but significantly increased pain means you should stop and seek help from a doctor. Even simple exhaustion is probably a sign that you're trying to do too much.

2. Does that mean that if my pain level increases a little after starting a new exercise regimen, it's normal?

It's normal to have a modest increase in discomfort or muscle soreness for the first three to four weeks after you start an exercise program. Any sharp stabbing pain or increase in pain overall means either your regimen is wrong for you or you need to consult your doctor.

3. My sciatic pain has increased and my leg feels weaker. What's causing that? What should I do?

Increasing weakness is cause for concern and should be checked by a doctor immediately. Your nerve inflammation may have increased for a number of reasons, and needs to be investigated.

4. I am having increased back pain with new symptoms of difficulty maintaining my urinary stream. What should I do?

This could be a real medical emergency. It may be a condition called cauda equina syndrome. You need to see a doctor immediately to rule it out.

5. I hear occasional pops and crackling in my arthritic joint. What is that?

It could be joint fluid coming out of your joint because your joint is producing too much fluid caused by inflammation. Icing the joint two or three times a day will help. However, most of the time it can be caused by minor variations in atmospheric pressure throughout the day. Decrease your overall level of inflammation by following my Stop Pain Regimen and that will help decrease the fluid production and thus the pops and crackling.

6. I have significant morning stiffness in my arthritic back and wrist, but then it gets better during the day. What should I do?

Morning stiffness in low back and/or joints in the wrist or hand that improves as the day goes on is a cause for concern. You must see a doctor to rule out autoimmune diseases such as rheumatoid arthritis.

7. The pain level in my arthritic knee joint goes up before it rains. Myth or reality?

Atmospheric pressure decreases a day or two before it rains. The joint has to adjust to atmospheric pressure. An arthritic joint trying to adjust will cause pain or discomfort. In the same way, your arthritic knee or back may become more inflamed when you fly on an airplane, because of the change in cabin pressure. Women may experience similar increases in pain levels during their menstrual period because of changes in hormonal activity.

8. I have pain in my shoulder or low back when I sleep. What could be the cause?

The most common cause of night shoulder pain is a full tear in your rotator cuff. The most common cause of night pain in the low back and/or leg is an inflamed nerve. Both conditions will cause pain whether or not you sleep on the affected area. Occasionally, especially for smokers, a cancer lesion could manifest as nighttime pain in the shoulder or low back. In the presence of night pain, you should see your doctor.

9. Are there any cautions about taking too many dietary supplements—especially vitamins A, E, and K, glucosamine, or ginger?

For people with diabetes, glucosamine could raise blood sugar levels, so check with your doctor before taking this. More than 510 milligrams daily of ginger could raise blood pressure or thin blood too much. Consult with your doctor if you are on blood pressure medication or blood thinners.

Vitamins A, E, and K are fat-based, unlike water-soluble vitamin C, so ingesting too much of these could give you vitamin toxicity. Also be careful when taking Chinese herbs or tea, as they may adversely affect the heart. Check with your doctor before using these.

10. Do different climates have an impact on arthritis pain?

In general, the colder and damper climates tend to exacerbate arthritis pain, whereas warmer and drier climates tend to have an ameliorating effect on joint pain. In my opinion it's largely because the warmer and drier climate has fewer variations in atmospheric pressure.

11. I have spinal stenosis that suddenly gets worse in the wintertime and feels better in warmer weather. Am I imagining this?

I often hear from my patients with spinal stenosis that it's symptomatic in colder months, less symptomatic in warmer months. But chronic pain syndromes such as spinal stenosis also tend to be cyclical, although no one is certain why this happens. The condition may go into quiet remission for several months or longer, then become active and painful again for some time before it once again mysteriously disappears. These cycles sometimes seem to be tied to the seasons, but again, we can't be certain. We also know that some people tend to get depressed in winter because of the shorter days and the lack of sunlight—a condition called seasonal affective disorder, or SAD. Because depression and pain are linked, it's possible that the changes in physical symptoms are indeed linked to the seasons.

Afterword

In my years of treating chronic pain, I have seen many changes in how people approach this journey to an enhanced quality of life. Our understanding of the physiological mechanisms that affect pain continues to advance. As you've seen, the link between inflammation and the nervous system has led to new insights on managing chronic pain. And exciting advances in treatment technology are happening on many fronts. For example, new MRI technology is able to detect such things as loss of cartilage in the knee joint or loss of hydration in discs in the low back at a very early stage. This early diagnosis will help doctors prescribe proper early treatments that will slow the natural progression of loss of cartilage, so people won't have to fight the pain of advanced stages of these conditions.

It seems also that future treatments will be more localized to avoid systemic side effects, and treatment materials will resemble biologic tissues, like the platelet-rich plasma described in Chapter Nine. Or the use of bone morphogenic proteins (BMPs), which induce the formation of bone and cartilage, to encourage bone growth instead of relying on metal inserts to surgically fuse the spine. Research is also underway at biotech companies investigating injectable gels that resemble our own joint fluid. The goal of repairing tears in spinal discs is being approached from a number of angles. Mobitech, a privately held biotech company I founded, is now investigating the role of stem cells, while other groups are looking at using gene therapy in an effort to repair painful tears in the disc.

The pharmaceutical world is investigating new ways to use nanotechnology to block pain without the negative side effects of narcotics. In the arena of OTC self-care options, companies are working to develop topical gels that relieve pain better and for longer duration. You'll see a wide assortment of patches on the market with newer materials like the hydrogels that the Inflasoothe Group and many other companies are working to develop.

Though financing for basic scientific research is limited, more and more funders are beginning to help. They see the importance of understanding the root of a problem in order to make the monumental leaps needed to treat pain. The Vad Foundation that I established in 2008 is now funding basic research into how arthritis develops. And many other foundations, including the Arthritis Foundation and the North American Spine Society, and governmental agencies such as the National Institutes of Health, are also funding basic science research.

Between our growing knowledge of pain and the emerging technologies that will help us diagnose and treat it, the future for chronic pain relief is very bright.

Appendix A

What to Do If You Are in Severe Acute Pain Right NOW

After an injury to your back or any joint or extremity, follow these basic steps to relieve your pain and begin healing.

1. Take 48 hours of modified bed rest. The body is designed to heal itself, but you have to give it time to concentrate on healing. Spend most of the day resting quietly in the position that you find most comfortable and soothing, depending on the nature of your injury. Lying on your back with both legs raised or with your knees supported by a pillow, for instance, helps your lower back muscles relax by taking the strain off them. You may also lie on one side with a pillow between your legs. Don't lie on your stomach if you have lower-back pain.

2. During this time you can get up every couple of hours to walk around, go to the bathroom, or eat. But don't do strenuous exercise, take long walks, or sit in a chair for more than a few minutes at a time.

3. During the first day or two of modified bed rest, you should apply ice three or four times a day, for 15 minutes

maximum to lessen inflammation. More than 15 minutes of ice will not provide additional benefits. You can apply a little compression (an elastic surgical bandage, such as an Ace bandage) and elevate the affected limb.

4. After the first day or two, begin applying heat in the morning and before any physical activity; use ice at bedtime or after activity, 10 to 15 minutes at a time. If your pain responds better to heat or to ice, adjust the sequence accordingly.

5. Apply The MD System oil or cream or Biofreeze to affected areas twice a day.

6. Take at least ten deep breaths through your nose three or four times a day. This not only shifts the mind away from the pain but also relaxes the body by stimulating the parasympathetic nervous system. The main actions of the parasympathetic nervous system are "rest and repose," in contrast to the fight-or-flight response of the sympathetic nervous system, which is stimulated by short, shallow breathing. Deep breathing also delivers added oxygen to overstressed, aching muscles and discs, which in turn allows them to relax and take in nourishment. Do this while seated in a chair or sitting up in bed, with arms and legs uncrossed. Breathe in as deeply as you can in a slow, steady rhythm but without straining. Hold your breath a few moments after each inhalation and exhalation. You should be able to feel your abdomen expand slightly on the inhale and contract again on the exhale. Each session of breathing should last at least two or three minutes, or more if you enjoy the calming sensation.

7. You may also visualize a white or golden light flowing into your body, from the crown of your head, down the spinal column, and out to your extremities. This will guide your breathing and help you relax even more.

8. If you still don't feel better, take three ibuprofen (Advil, Motrin, or generic) twice a day as long as you don't have any medical issues, such as ulcers or kidney damage. Check with your doctor if you have diabetes, as even a dose this small can have bad effects on the kidneys of people with diabetes. Ibuprofen combines pain relief with an anti-inflammatory effect and is generally more beneficial for acute pain than acetaminophen. If they don't give you any significant relief after two or three days, see a doctor, who can prescribe more powerful pain relievers, anti-inflammatories, or muscle relaxants. These are safe for a limited period of time if taken as directed. If you still get no relief after several days, consult again with your physician for other alternatives.

Appendix B

Sample Exercises for Low-Back Strength and Treating Arthritis of the Hip and Knee

The following exercises are taken from my books and DVDs entitled *Back Rx* and *Arthritis Rx*. For complete exercise routines, please refer to those books and DVDs, available through www.vijayvad.com and most online booksellers.

STRETCHES FOR LOW-BACK STRENGTH

Hip Internal Rotation Stretch

This is designed to increase hip flexibility to take the load off the low back

- Lie on your back with your arms stretched out to your sides and palms on the floor.

- Bending both knees, place your right foot flat on the floor in front of you.

- Then cross your left leg over your right thigh and gently allow its weight to pull your right leg toward the floor.

- Hold 10 seconds.

- Repeat 3 times each side

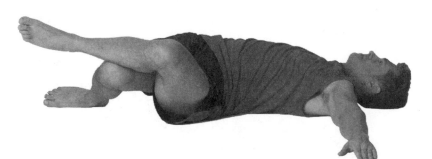

Abdominal Crunch

This exercise is designed to strengthen the abdominals, which, in turn, stabilize your low back.

- Lie on your back with arms at your sides and palms flat on the floor.

- Slowly raise each knee to a bent position, keeping feet flat on the floor, and put your hands behind your head.

- Inhale deeply through your nose as you raise your shoulders slightly from the floor and squeeze your abs. Keep your hands behind your head to minimize pressure on the neck, but don't pull your head. Just keep your neck straight and let your head follow your shoulders off the floor.

- Exhale through your mouth, then hold for at least 10 seconds while continuing to breathe deeply 3 or 4 times.

- Repeat 2 more times.

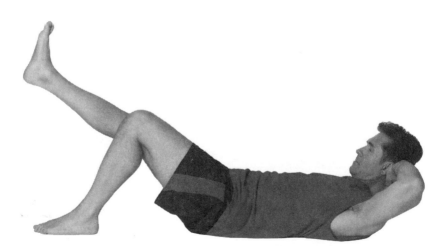

Tree Pose

This pose derived from yoga will help you develop balance and core strength for good back health.

- Stand straight and tall with your feet nearly together—the outer edge of your big toes should be touching, but your heels should be separated slightly. Stand up straight with your eyes looking directly in front of you, as if at a distant horizon.

- Angle one leg outward, and bring the heel of the foot up to rest on the inside of your other leg above or below the knee. Avoid putting your foot directly at your knee, as that applies unnecessary pressure to your knee joint. If that's too difficult, then simply angle your knee outward as if you were going to complete the pose, but only lift your heel—leave your toes on the ground.

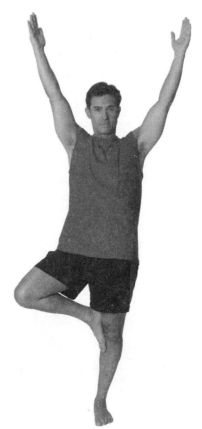

- Inhale slowly through your nose as you raise your arms to reach for the sky.

- Exhale slowly through your nose, and take two more deep breaths in and out.

- Relax to the starting position as you take a fourth full breath.

- Repeat two more times, then switch to the other leg and follow the same procedure.

STRETCHES FOR ARTHRITIS OF KNEE AND HIP

Iliotibial Band (ITB) and Hip Stretch

Use this stretch to help restore the proper biomechanics of hip and knee, and increase the stretch of the ITB and the paraspinal muscles.

- Sit on the floor with your back erect and your legs straight in front of you and flat on the floor.

- Now, bend and raise your right knee, cross your right leg over your left and place your right foot flat on the floor alongside your left knee and parallel to your left leg, with your toes pointed forward.

- Twist your shoulders and upper torso toward the right and place your left elbow on the outside of your right knee.

- Push your right knee toward the left with your left elbow as you continue to rotate your upper torso to the right until you feel the stretch deep in your right buttock.

- Keep your back straight and erect. Hold the stretch for 10 seconds.

- Repeat twice more, then reverse everything to stretch the left leg.

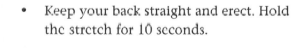

Hip-Strengthening Exercise

Designed to strengthen hip musculature along with developing balance.

- Hold your arms straight out in front of you and parallel to each other, palms facing down.

- Lift right leg to the side so that all your weight is on the left leg.

- Hold 10 seconds.

- Repeat 2 more times.

- Replace right leg on the floor, lift left leg and hold 10 seconds.

- Repeat twice more.

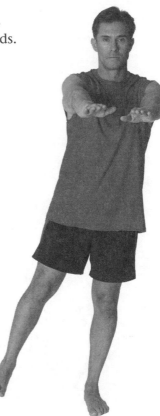

Cross-Leg Stretch

This stretch is designed to increase flexibility in the hip and stretch the low back.

- Stand with legs wider apart than your shoulders.

- Bending forward, gently stretch to touch the toes of your right foot with your left fingertips.

- Hold for 10 seconds.

- Repeat twice more.

- Repeat the series three times with your right hand touching your left foot.

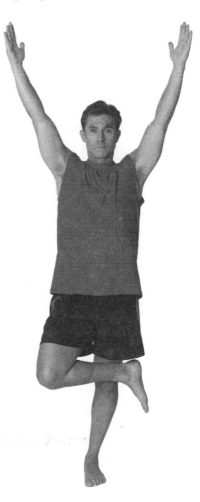

Appendix C

Resources

MEDICAL SUPPLIES AND EQUIPMENT

Pneumatic Armband by Aircast

I recommend that my patients with tennis elbow use the Pneumatic Armband to apply compression where it is needed, while lessening the constriction of uninvolved muscles and blood flow.

Aircast DJO, LLC
1430 Decision Street
Vista, CA 92081
800-336-6569
www.aircast.com

Brookstone

Although it's not a medical supply company, Brookstone makes some of the best gear for travel comfort, especially neck rests like the Tempur-Pedic Transit Pillow and an assortment of sleep masks that help you rest comfortably on long flights. I also recommend their NapForm Eye Mask to help ensure sound sleep at home by blocking out all ambient light.

800-846-3000
www.brookstone.com/travel-comfort-products.html

CryoTherm

Corflex makes a wide selection of CryoTherm gel packs and other products, including E/N lumbar supports and shoulder wraps that are among the best you can find anywhere. The majority of my patients with chronic back pain rank the compression wrap with the cold gel pack as one of the top three things that have helped them the most.

Corflex
669 East Industrial Park Drive
Manchester, NH 03109
603-623-3344
www.corflex.com

Disc Unloader Brace (Disc Unloader Orthosis)

I personally designed this device to take pressure off the low back. In clinical trials, the brace has been shown to reduce pressure between discs by 40 percent while sitting, with significant pain reduction. (The brace is being prescribed nationally by my colleagues and was mentioned as one of the best-designed braces for treating low-back pain by the Wall Street Journal in 2005.) The brace is available by prescription for those with chronic disc pain who are unable to sit for long periods of time.

Corflex
603-623-3344
www.corflex.com

Lifecore Straight Back Recumbent Bicycle

Recumbent bikes are ideal for those who suffer from arthritis of the hip, knee, or ankle but still want the aerobic workout provided by bicycling without putting undue pressure on the joints. Lifecore makes some of the best recumbent bikes, and my favorite is the LC-1000RB

Lifecore Fitness
2575 Pioneer Avenue, #101
Vista, CA 92081
888-815-5559
www.lifecorefitness.com

Wal-Pil-O Pillow

This is the best ergonomic pillow I have experienced. It offers several different-sized edges so you can find the appropriate size to cradle your neck and head, providing proper support and alignment whether you sleep on your back or side. It also comes in an air pump-up version for more adjustable fit.

The Wal-Pil-O Store
A division of Pain Reliever Stores
888-498-8587
www.WalPiloStore.com

WellPatch

Use WellPatch Pain Relieving Pads for sustained heat during the workday. They adhere to your body and are thin and flexible enough to wear under your clothes; they're also greaseless and odorless, so you can wear them at work without anyone noticing. WellPatch Heat Warming Pads work the same way to apply heat that can help alleviate minor aches, pains and stiffness in muscles and joints. Using these heat patches during the day followed by icing the back with the Corflex compression wrap after work is one of the most effective combinations I know for treating chronic pain.

The Mentholatum Co.
707 Sterling Drive
Orchard Park, New York 14127
877-636-2677
www.wellpatch.com

DIETARY SUPPLEMENTS, CAPSULES, TABLETS, AND OILS

Barlean's Organic Oils

An excellent source of unrefined, unfiltered flaxseed oil as well as omega oil blends produced without destructive heating methods.

4936 Lake Terrell Road
Ferndale, Washington 98248
800-445-3529
www.barleans.com

Twinlab

Twinlab makes one of the best omega-3 EFA blends. Their Mega Twin EPA/DHA softgels are derived from deep-sea, cold-water fish and screened to avoid toxic elements present in some deep-sea fish, such as PCBs and heavy metals.

Ideasphere, Inc.
600 East Quality Drive
American Fork, UT 84003
800-645-5626
www.twinlab.com

Gingerflex

Taken as directed, my personally designed product supplies the recommended amounts of glucosamine sulfate (1,500 milligrams), condroitin (1,200 milligrams), and ginger (510 milligrams) for relief of arthritis pain.

877-8-GINGER

www.gingerflex.com

Country Life Vitamins

Vitamin D3 from non-fish liver sources, available in 2,500 and 5,000 IU softgels.

180 Vanderbilt Motor Parkway

Hauppauge, NY 11788

800-645-5768

www.countrylifevitamins.com

Nutramax Laboratories, Inc.

Makers of Cosamin-DS, the brand of glucosamine sulfate and condroitin on which the New England Journal of Medicine trials were done. It is reliable and pure.

2208 Lakeside Boulevard

Edgewood, MD 21040

888-886-6442

www.nutramaxlabs.com

Nature's Plus

As far as I know, their Ultra Bromelain is the only version of this valuable enzyme available in 1,500 milligrams tablets. Take one a day to help relieve MSK pain.

Natural Organics Laboratories
Amityville, NY 11701
www.naturesplus.com

Nature's Way

Their products include a wide range of reliable herbal supplements in powder form for those who don't like to use tinctures, especially when traveling.

800-9NATURE
www.naturesway.com

Mountain Naturals of Vermont

20 New England Drive, Suite 10
Essex Junction, VT 05452
800-992-8451
www.mountainnaturals.com

Nordic Naturals

Noted for their omega-3 fish oil supplements.

94 Hangar Way
Watsonville, CA 95076
800-662-2544 x1
www.nordicnaturals.com

TINCTURES

Quantum Herbal Products

20 Dewitt Drive
Saugerties, NY 12477
845-246-1344
www.quantumherbalproducts.com

Herbal Remedies

322 7th Avenue
New York, NY 10001
USA: 866-467-6444 or worldwide: 1-212-279-4351
www.herbalremedies.com

TOPICALS, CREAMS, AND GELS

The MD System

Created by the Inflasoothe Group, clinical trials of this system were done in May 2009. Of those subjects using the oil 15 minutes before playing golf, 64 percent had statistically significant pain relief compared to placebo, and 70 percent reported good or excellent satisfaction. A version of this topical is now being made available commercially without a prescription as The MD System cream and high-strength oil.

www.TheMDSystem.com

Biofreeze

This pain-relieving gel, available from a tube, pump bottle, or roll-on, has proven effective in the temporary relief of joint and muscle pain from arthritis, bursitis, and other MSK ailments.

Performance Health
2230 Boyd Road
Export, PA 15632
800-246-3733

Zostrix

Effective analgesic cream comes in regular and high-potency formulas, as well as a neuropathy cream to treat diabetic foot pain.

Hi Tech Pharmacal Co.
369 Bayview Avenue
Amityville, NY 11701
800-899-3116
www.zostrix.com

Aspercreme

This topical salicylate pain reliever, available as a cream, lotion, or gel, works by reducing swelling and inflammation in muscles and joints. Its active ingredient is derived from salicylic acid, much like aspirin—hence the brand name.

Bengay

Popular analgesic heat rub used to relieve muscle and joint pain was developed in France and brought to America in 1898 (spelled Ben-Gay prior to 1995).

Capzasin-P

The active ingredient in this topical, which comes in several forms, is capsaicin (derived from hot chili peppers). Although we're not certain, capsaicin is believed to moderate the flow of substance P, which transmits pain sensations.

GRASS-FED MEAT

Eatwild

The most comprehensive source for grass-fed meat and dairy products in the United States and Canada; lists more than 1,100 pasture-based farms that produce beef, lamb, pork, bison, and other meats.

USA: 866-453-8489, or worldwide: 253-759-2318
www.eatwild.com

PAIN TREATMENT

American Academy of Pain Management

An organization for professionals working with people in pain, the AAPM provides accreditation, continuing education, publications, and other services.

209-533-9744
www.aapainmanage.org

American Chronic Pain Association

This organization and the following one provide information, advocacy, and support for chronic pain sufferers and their families.

800-533-3231
www.theacpa.org

American Pain Foundation

www.painfoundation.org
888-665-PAIN (7246)

National Foundation for the Treatment of Pain

Provides comprehensive information and referrals to pain specialists.

916-725-5669
www.paincare.org

Endnotes

INTRODUCTION

1. "In 1999 MarketdataEnterprises estimated that approximately 4.9 million Americans saw a physician for chronic pain." Pain Management Programs: A market Analysis, MarketdataEnterprises, 1999, Tampa, Florida.

   Chronic Pain in America: Roadblocks to relief, survey conducted for the American Pain Society, The American Academy of Pain Medicine and Janssen Pharmaceutica, 1999.

   American Pain Foundation, www.painfoundation.org/learn/publications/files/PainFactsandStats.pdf

2. B.M. Kuehn, "Opioid prescriptions soar: increase in legitimate use as well as abuse." *JAMA* 297 (2007): 249–251.

3. American Sports Data, Inc., americansportsdata.com/obesitystats.asp G. Affleck, S. Urrows, H. Tennen, P. Higgins, and M. Abeles, "Sequential daily relations of sleep, pain intensity, and attention to pain among women with fibromyalgia," *Pain* 68 (1996): 363–368. Abstract.

4. Thomas Roth, PhD, "The Impact of Disturbed Sleep on Pain," Medscape Today, medscape.com/viewarticle/506217.

CHAPTER ONE

1. Nicolas E. Walsh, Peter Brooks, J. Mieke Hazes, Rorey M. Walsh, Karsten Dreinhofer, Anthony D. Woolf, Kristina Akesson, and Lars Lidgren, for the Bone and Joint Decade Task Force for Standards of Care for Acute and Chronic Musculoskeletal Pain, "Standards of Care for Acute and Chronic Musculoskeletal Pain: The Bone and Joint Decade (2000–2010)," *Arch Phys Med Rehabil,* 89 (Sept. 2008): 1830–1845.

2. Stephanie Clipper (NINDS), "What Causes Pain," MentalHelp.net, www.mentalhelp.net/poc/view_doc.php?type=doc&id=4688&cn=81.

3. René Descartes, *L'homme de René Descartes*, Paris: Charles Angot, 1664, cited in Melzack and Wall, 1983, p.196.

4. H.K. Beecher, *Measurement of Subjective Responses* (New York: Oxford University Press, 1959).

CHAPTER THREE

1. Center for Disease Control and Prevention reports on chronic fatigue syndrome, www.cdc.gov/cfs.

2. Zivadinov et al., "Epstein-Barr Virus is Associated with Gray Matter Atrophy in Multiple Sclerosis," *Journal of Neurology Neurosurgery & Psychiatry*; DOI: 10.1136/jnnp.2008.154906.

3. S.E. Straus, G. Tosato, G. Armstrong, T. Lawley, et al., "Persisting illness and fatigue in adults, with evidence of Epstein-Barr infection." *Annals of Internal Medicine* 102 (1985): 7–16.

4. D. Buchwald, J.L. Sullivan, A.L. Komaroff, "Frequency of 'chronic active Epstein-Barr' virus infection in a general medical practice," *JAMA* 257 (1987): 2303–2307.

5. G.P. Holmes, J.E. Kaplan, J.A. Stewart, et al., "A cluster of patients with a chronic mononucleosis-like syndrome" *JAMA* 257 (1987): 2297–2302.

CHAPTER FOUR

1. George Mateljan, "Open Letter to President Barack Obama," June 24, 2009, http://whfoods.org/genpage.php?tname=george&dbid=249.

2. Michal Toborek, Yong Woo Lee, Rosario Garrido, Simone Kaiser, and Bernhard Hennig. "Unsaturated fatty acids selectively induce an inflammatory environment in human endothelial cells." *American Journal of Clinical Nutrition*, 75, No. 1 (January 2002): 119–125.

3. Eunyoung Cho, Johanna M. Seddon, Bernard Rosner, Walter C. Willett, and Susan E. Hankinson, "Prospective Study of Intake of Fruits, Vegetables, Vitamins, and Carotenoids and Risk of Age-Related Maculopathy," *Arch Ophthalmol*, 122 (2004): 883–892.

4. W. Gifford Jones, "The Anti-Inflammatory Diet: A Diet for All Ages," *Canada Free Press*, March 1, 2005, canadafreepress.com/medical/cardio-vascular030105.htm.

5. "What You Need to Know About Mercury in Fish and Shellfish," EPA-823-R-04-005, March 2004, www.cfsan.fda.gov/~dms/admehg3.html. See also "Mercury Levels in Commercial Fish and Shellfish," updated Feb. 2006.

6. Je-Ruei Lin, Ming-Ju Chen, and Chin-Win Lin, "Antimutagenic and Antioxidant Properties of Milk-Kefir and Soymilk-Kefir," *Journal of Agricultural and Food Chemistry* 53 No. 7 (2005): 2467–2474.

   Elena Conis, "Kefir is nutritious, but larger health claims are on shakier ground," *The Los Angeles Times*, Sept. 15, 2008.

7. According to figures compiled by the Mayo Clinic. Dietary Fiber chart available online at: www.mayoclinic.com/health/high-fiber-foods/NU00582.

CHAPTER FIVE

1. Vijay B. Vad, A.L. Bhat, and Y. Tarabichi, "The Role of the Back RX Exercise Program in diskogenic low back pain: A prospective randomized trial, *Arch Phys Med Rehabil*, 88 (May 2007): 577–582.

2. L.E. Armstrong, D.J. Casa, C.M.Maresh, M.S. Ganio "Caffeine, fluid-electrolyte balance, temperature regulation, and exercise-heat tolerance," *Exerc. Sport Sci. Rev.* 35(3) (2007): 135–140. Doi:10.1097/jes.0b013e3180a02cc1. PMID 17620932.

   L.E. Armstrong, A.C. Pumerantz, M.W. Roti, D.A. Judelson, G. Watson, J.C. Dias, B. Sokmen, D.J. Casa, C.M. Maresh, H.Lieberman, and M. Kellogg, "Fluid, electrolyte, and renal indices of hydration during 11 days of controlled caffeine consumption," Int. *J. Sport Nutr. Exerc. Metab.* 15(3) (2005): 252–265. PMID 16131696.

3. Melissa Walker, "Endorphins 101: Your Guide to Natural Euphoria." Online at http://yourtotalhealth.ivillage.com/endorphins-101-your-guide-natural-euphoria.html.

4. Melissa Conrad Stoppler, "Endorphins: Natural Pain and Stress Fighters," medicinenet.com/script/main/art.asp?articlekey=55001.

5. Jeremy S. Sibold, and Kathy Berg, University of Vermont, Burlington, "Mood Enhancement Persists for up to 12 Hours Following Aerobic Exercise," American College of Sports Medicine 56th Annual Meeting, May 27, 2009.

6. Roni Cary Rabin, "Alcohol Is Good for You? Some Scientists Doubt It." *The New York Times,* June 16, 2009.

7. Ibid.

CHAPTER SEVEN

1. Memorial Sloan-Kettering: www.mskcc.org/mskcc/html/ 11570.cfm. National Institutes of Health: www.nlm.nih.gov/ medlineplus/druginfo/herb_All.html#B.

2. Omega-3 oils and Oleocanthol:

    Gary K. Beauchamp, Russell S.J. Keast, Diane Morel, Jianming Lin, Jana Pika, Qiang Han, Chi-Ho Lee, Amos B. Smith, and Paul A.S. Breslin, "Phytochemistry: Ibuprofen-like activity in extra-virgin olive oil." *Nature* 437(7055) (2005): 45–46.

    M.W. Whitehouse and D.E. Butters, "Combination anti-inflammatory therapy: synergism in rats of NSAIDs / corticosteroids with some herbal / animal products," *Inflammopharmacology* 11(4–6) (2003): 453–464.

3. Ginger:

    S. Phillips et al., "Zingiber officinale (ginger): An antiemetic for day case surgery," *Anaesthesia* 48 (1993): 715–717.

    H. Kikuzaki and N. Nakatani, "Antioxidant effects of some ginger constituents," *J Food Science* 58 (1993): 1407.

    Y.B. Lee et al., "Antioxidant property in ginger rhizome and its application to meat products," *J Food Science* 51(1) (1986): 20–23.

    K.C. Srivastava and T. Mustafa, "Ginger (Zingiber officinale) and rheumatic disorders," *Med Hypotheses* 29(1) (May 1989): 25–28.

    K.C. Srivastava and T. Mustafa, "Ginger (Zingiber offincinale) in rheumatic and musculoskeletal disorders," *Med Hypotheses* 39(4) (Dec. 1992): 342–348.

R. Altman and K.C. Marcussen, "Effects of ginger on knee pain in patients with osteoarthritis," *Arthritis and Rheumatism* 44(11) (2001): 2531–2538.

I. Wigler, I. Grotto, D. Caspi, and M. Yaron, "The effects of Zintona EC (a ginger extract) on symptomatic gonarthritis," *Osteoarthritis Cartilage*, 11(11) (Nov. 2003): 783–789.

4.   Glucosamine and Condroitine Sulfate:

E. Ernst, V.S. Vassiliou, J.-P. Pelletier, D.O. Clegg, and D.J. Reda, "Glucosamine and Chondroitin Sulfate for Knee Osteoarthritis," *New England Journal of Medicine* 354 (May 18, 2006): 2184–2185.

J.Y. Reginster, "Long term effects of glucosamine sulfate on osteoarthritis progression: A randomized, placebo-controlled trial," *Lancet* 357 (2001): 251–256.

A. Kahan, et al. "Long-term effects of condroitin sulfate on knee osteoarthritis," *Arthritis & Rheumatism* 60 (2009): 524–533.

5.   Flavonoids:

R. Levy, R. Saikovsky, E. Shmidt, and A. Khokhlov, "Safety, efficacy and acceptability of flavocoxid (Limbrelcom) compared with naproxen in subjects with osteoarthritis of the knee: a pilot study," *Osteoarthritis and Cartilage* 15(suppl B) (2007): B91.

Donald R. Buhler and Miranda Cristobal, "Antioxidant Activities of Flavonoids," Department of Environmental and Molecular Toxicology, Oregon State University, http://lpi.oregonstate.edu/f-w00/flavonoid.html.

S.B. Lotito and B. Frei, "Consumption of flavonoid-rich foods and increased plasma antioxidant capacity in humans: cause, consequence, or epiphenomenon?" *Free Radic Biol Med.* 41 (2006): 1727–1746.

P. Galley and M. Thiollet, "A double-blind, placebo-controlled trial of a new veno-active flavonoid fraction (S 5682) in the treatment of symptomatic capillary fragility," *Int Angiol* 12 (1993): 69–72.

D. Bagchi, C.K. Sen, S.D. Ray, et al., "Molecular mechanisms of cardioprotection by a novel grape seed proanthocyanidin extract," *Mutat Res.* 523–524 (Feb.-March 2003): 87–97. PMID 12628506.

O. Vitseva, S. Varghese, S. Chakrabarti, J.D. Folts, and J.E. Freedman, "Grape seed and skin extracts inhibit platelet function and release of reactive oxygen intermediates," *J Cardiovasc Pharmacol.* 46(4) (Oct. 2005): 445–451. doi:10.1097/01.fjc.0000176727.67066.1c. PMID 16160595.

J.K. Kundu and Y.J. Surh "Cancer chemopreventive and therapeutic potential of resveratrol: mechanistic perspectives," *Cancer Lett.* 269(2) (Oct. 2008): 243–261. doi:10.1016/j.canlet.2008.03.057. PMID 18550275.

University of California, Davis—Health System, "Study Shows Grape Seed Extract May Be Effective In Reducing Blood Pressure." *Science Daily* 27 (March 2006). ww.sciencedaily.com/releases/2006/03/060327084242.htm.

6. Boswellia:

U. Dahmen, Y.L.Gu, O. Dirsch, et al. "Boswellic acid, a potent anti-inflammatory drug, inhibits rejection to the same extent as high dose steroids," *Transplant Proc.* 33(1-2) (Feb.-March 2001): 539–541.

H. Safayhi, S.E. Boden, S. Schweizer, et al., "Concentration-dependent potentiating and inhibitory effects of Boswellia extracts on 5-lipoxygenase product formation in stimulated PMNL," *Planta Med.* 66(2) (March 2000): 110–113.

I. Gupta, V. Gupta, A. Parihar, et al., "Effects of Boswellia serrata gum resin in patients with bronchial asthma: results of a double-blind, placebo-controlled, 6-week clinical study," *European Journal of Herbal Medicine* 3 (1998): 511–514.

7. Bromelain:

Commission E is an authoritative committee of physicians, pharmacists, medical researchers and toxicologists created by the German government in 1978 to monitor the effectiveness and safety of German herbal medicine for treatment of sinusitis, postsurgical inflammation and pain, and post-traumatic athletic injuries.

Michael Heinrich,, A.D. Kinghorn, and J.D. Phillipson, *Fundamentals of Pharmacognosy and Phytotherapy* (Churchill Livingstone, 2004) p. 265.

D.J. Fitzhugh, S. Shan, M.W. Dewhirst, et al., "Bromelain treatment decreases neutrophil migration to sites of inflammation," *Clinical Immunology* 128 (2008): 66–74.

A.F. Walker, et al. "Bromelain reduces mild acute knee pain and improves well-being in a dose-dependent fashion in an open study of otherwise healthy adults," *Phytomedicine* 9(8) (Dec. 2002): 681–686.

S. Brien, G. Lewith, A.F. Walker, et al., "Bromelain as an adjunctive treatment for moderate-to-severe osteoarthritis of the knee: a randomized, placebo-controlled pilot study," *QJM* 99(12) (Dec. 2006): 841–850.

G. Klein, W. Kullich, J. Schnitker, et al., "Efficacy and tolerance of an oral enzyme combination in painful osteoarthritis of the hip. A double-blind, randomised study comparing oral enzymes with non-steroidal anti-inflammatory drugs," *Clin Exp Rheumatol.* 24(1) (Jan.–Feb. 2006): 25–30.

8. Resveratrol:

Mayo Clinic Online, www.mayoclinic.com/health/red-wine/ HB00089.

B. Fauconneau et al., "Comparative study of radical scavenger and antioxidant properties of phenolic compounds from Vitis vinifera cell cultures using in vitro tests." *Life Sci* 61(21) (1997): 2103–2110.

C.R. Pace-Asciak et al., "The red wine phenolics trans-resveratrol and quercetin block human platelet aggregation and eicosanoid synthesis: implications for protection against coronary heart disease," *Clin Chim Acta* 235(2) (1995): 207–219.

S.V. Culpitt et al., "Inhibition by red wine extract, resveratrol, of cytokine release by alveolar macrophages in COPD," *Thorax* 58(11) (2003): 942–946.

9. MSM:

P.R. Usha and M.U.R. Naidu, "Randomised, double-blind, parallel, placebo-controlled study of oral glucosamine, methylsulfonylmethane and their combination in osteoarthritis," *Clin Drug Invest* 24(6) (2004): 353–363

L.S. Kim, L.J. Axelrod, P. Howard, N. Buratovich, and R.F. Waters, "Efficacy of methylsulfonylmethane (MSM) in osteoarthritis pain of the knee: a pilot clinical trial," *Osteoarthritis Cartilage* 14(3) (2006): 286–294. PMID 16309928.

10. Vitamin D3:

Michael F. Holick, "Vitamin D Deficiency," *NEJM* 357(3) (July 19, 2007): 266–281. www.nejm.org.

Lee, et al., "Association between 25-hydroxyvitamin D levels and cognitive performance in middle-aged and older European men,"

Journal of Neurology, Neurosurgery and Psychiatry, 2009. DOI: 10.1136/jnnp.2008.165720.

Y. Agrawal, J.P. Carey, C.C. Della Santina, M.C. Schubert, and L.B. Minor, "Disorders of balance and vestibular function in U.S. adults: data from the National Health and Nutrition Examination Survey, 2001-2004." *Arch Intern Med.* 169(10) (May 25, 2009): 938–944.

S. Muthayya, A. Eilander, C. Transler, T. Thomas, H.C.M. van der Knaap, et al., "Effect of fortification with multiple micronutrients and n–3 fatty acids on growth and cognitive performance in Indian schoolchildren: the CHAMPION (Children's Health and Mental Performance Influenced by Optimal Nutrition) Study," *Am J Clin Nutr.* 89 (2009): 1766–1775.

"Exeter research links 'sunshine vitamin' to cognitive problems in older people." University of Exeter online at www.exeter.ac.uk/research/excellence/keythemes/medicine/news/title,2176,en.php.

CHAPTER NINE

1. V. Vad et al., "Transforaminal Epidural Steroid Injections in Lumbosacral Radiculopathy: A Prospective Randomized Study," *Spine* 27 (2002): 11–16.

2. P. Dreyfuss, et al., "Efficacy and Validity of Lumbar Medial Branch Radiofrequency Neurotomy for Chronic Zygapophyseal Joint Pain," *Spine* 25 (2000): 1270–1277.

3. A. Mishra and T. Pavelko, "Treatment of chronic elbow tendinosis with buffered platelet-rich plasma," *Am J.Sports Med* (2006): 1774–1778.

CHAPTER TEN

1. D.M. Eisenberg et al., "Unconventional Medicine in the United States," *NEJM* 328(4) (Jan. 28, 1993): 246–252.

Sita Ananth, "CAM: An Increasing Presence in U.S. Hospitals," Hospitals & Health Networks, online at www.hhnmag.com/hhnmag.

2. E. Ernst, "Chiropractic: a critical evaluation," *Journal of Pain Symptom Management*, 35(5) (May 2008): 544–562. Epub 2008 Feb. 14, MedLine.

3. D.C. Cherkin, et al., "A review of the evidence for the effectiveness, safety, and cost of acupuncture, massage therapy, and spinal manipulation for back pain," *Annals of Internal Medicine* 138(11) (2003): 898–907.

4. "Acupuncture—Consensus Development Conference Statement," NIH Consensus Development Program (Nov. 3–5, 1997), National Institutes of Health. http://consensus.nih. gov/1997/1997Acupuncture107html.htm.

5. Ibid

6. B.M. Berman, et al., "Effectiveness of Acupuncture as adjunctive therapy in osteoarthritis of the knee: a randomized, controlled trial," *Annals of Internal Medicine*, 141(12) (2004): 901–910.

7. National Center for Complementary and Alternative Medicine, National Institutes of Health, http://nccam.nih.gov/health/ acupuncture/introduction.htm#key.

CHAPTER ELEVEN

1. Daniel Goleman, "Relaxation: Surprising Benefits Detected," *The New York Times*, May 13, 1986.

2. HolisticOnline.com, available online at www.holisticonline.com/ remedies/Anxiety/anx_relaxation-response.htm.

3. "Depression and pain," Harvard Health Publications, https://www.health.harvard.edu/newsweek/Depression_and _pain.htm.

4. Daniel K. Hall-Flavin, "'Clinical' depression: What does that mean?" http://www.mayoclinic.com/health/clinical-depression/AN01057.

5. Harvard Health Publications, *op. cit.*

6. M.J. Sullivan, K. Reesor, S. Mikail, R. Fisher, "The treatment of depression in chronic low back pain: review and recommendations," *Pain* 50 (1992): 5–13.

7. Michael Clark "Managing Chronic Pain, Depression & Antidepressants: Issues & Relationships," www.hopkinsarthritis.org/ patient-corner/disease-management/depression.html.

M.E. Geisser, R.S. Roth, M.E. Theisen, et al., "Negative affect, self-report of depressive symptoms, and clinical depression: relation to the experience of chronic pain," *Clin J Pain* 16 (2000): 110–120.

CHAPTER TWELVE

1. Ray Sahelian, http://www.raysahelian.com/gaba.html.

Selected Bibliography

Cailliet, Rene. *Pain: Mechanisms and Management.*.Philadelphia: F.A. Davis Co., 1993.

Cordain, Loren. *The Paleo Diet: Lose Weight and Get Healthy by Eating the Food You Were Designed to Eat,* Hoboken, N.J.: Wiley, 2002.

Fors, Greg. *Why We Hurt: Your Total Self-Care Guide for Backaches, Headaches, Shoulder Pain, Arthritis and Fibromyalgia.* Woodbury, Minn.: Llewellyn Publications, 2007.

Gladstar, Rosemary. *Rosemary Gladstar's Family Herbal: A Guide to Living Life with Energy, Health, and Vitality.* North Adams, Mass.: Storey Books, 2001.

Heinerman, John. *Heinerman's Encyclopedia of Fruits, Vegetables, and Herbs.* Englewood Cliffs, N.J.: Prentice Hall, 1988.

Jensen, Bernard. *Foods That Heal: A Guide to Understanding and Using the Healing Powers of Natural Foods.* New York: Avery, 1993.

Leung, Albert and Steven Foster. *Encyclopedia of Common Natural Ingredients Used in Foods, Drugs, and Cosmetics.* New York: John Wiley & Sons, 1996.

Lipman, Frank with Mollie Doyle, *Spent: End Exhaustion and Feel Great Again.* New York: Fireside, 2009.

McGuffin,Michael,Christopher Hobbs, Roy Upton, and Alicia Goldberg, eds. *American Herbal Products Association's Botanical Safety Handbook*. CRC Press, 1997.

McMahon, Stephen & Martin Koltzenburg, eds. *Wall and Melzack's Textbook of Pain*, 5th ed. Churchill Livingstone, 2005.

Melzack, Ronald and Patrick D. Wall. *The Challenge of Pain*, revised ed., New York: Basic Books, 1983.

Index

Note: Page numbers in *italics* include illustrations and photographs.

Acknowledgments

I would like to thank Peter Occhiogrosso for his brilliant writing skills and compassion. I also want to thank Richard LaMotta for impressing upon me the need for inventing simple products for pain relief, and Maureen Taylor for convincing me that creating a book linking inflammation to pain is essential. I have had the privilege of working with an outstanding publishing company at Hay House, with a supportive and talented team in Patty Gift, Laura Koch, and Reid Tracy. Thanks also to Eric Angeloch for his artistic illustrations, and to Gloria Appel for her insightful suggestions. And finally a gracious thanks to Chris Godek, who has always given me golden advice, whether in publishing or in life.

About the Author

Vijay Vad, M.D., is a sports-medicine specialist at the Hospital for Special Surgery and a professor at Weill Medical College of Cornell University. He is the author of *Back Rx* and *Arthritis Rx*. In 2007, he created the Vad Foundation, dedicated to two causes: supporting medical research into back pain and arthritis, and funding education for disadvantaged girls worldwide. He co-founded The Inflasoothe Group in 2008. Dr. Vad lives in New York City with his wife, Dilshaad, and their children, Amoli and Nikhil.

Hay House Titles of Related Interest

YOU CAN HEAL YOUR LIFE, the movie,
starring Louise L. Hay & Friends
(available as a 1-DVD program and an expanded 2-DVD set)
Watch the trailer at: **www.LouiseHayMovie.com**

THE SHIFT, the movie, starring Dr. Wayne W. Dyer
(available as a 1-DVD program and an expanded 2-DVD set)
Watch the trailer at: **www.DyerMovie.com**

—

*COMMIT TO SIT: Tools for Cultivating a
Meditation Practice,* from the pages of *Tricycle* magazine;
edited by Joan Duncan Oliver

OM YOGA IN A BOX: The Basics, by Cyndi Lee

*THE VITAMIN D REVOLUTION: How the Power of This
Amazing Vitamin Can Change Your Life,* by Soram Khalsa, M.D.

YOU CAN HEAL YOUR LIFE, by Louise L. Hay

All of the above are available at your local bookstore,
or may be ordered by contacting Hay House (see next page).

We hope you enjoyed this Hay House book. If you'd like to receive our online catalog featuring additional information on Hay House books and products, or if you'd like to find out more about the Hay Foundation, please contact:

Hay House, Inc., P.O. Box 5100, Carlsbad, CA 92018-5100

(760) 431-7695 or (800) 654-5126
(760) 431-6948 (fax) or (800) 650-5115 (fax)
www.hayhouse.com® • www.hayfoundation.org

—

Published and distributed in Australia by: Hay House Australia Pty. Ltd., 18/36 Ralph St., Alexandria NSW 2015 • *Phone:* 612-9669-4299 *Fax:* 612-9669-4144 • www.hayhouse.com.au

Published and distributed in the United Kingdom by: Hay House UK, Ltd., 292B Kensal Rd., London W10 5BE • *Phone:* 44-20-8962-1230 *Fax:* 44-20-8962-1239 • www.hayhouse.co.uk

Published and distributed in the Republic of South Africa by: Hay House SA (Pty), Ltd., P.O. Box 990, Witkoppen 2068 • *Phone/Fax:* 27-11-467-8904 info@hayhouse.co.za • www.hayhouse.co.za

Published in India by: Hay House Publishers India, Muskaan Complex, Plot No. 3, B-2, Vasant Kunj, New Delhi 110 070 • *Phone:* 91-11-4176-1620 *Fax:* 91-11-4176-1630 • www.hayhouse.co.in

Distributed in Canada by: Raincoast, 9050 Shaughnessy St., Vancouver, B.C. V6P 6E5 • *Phone:* (604) 323-7100 *Fax:* (604) 323-2600 • www.raincoast.com

—

Take Your Soul on a Vacation

Visit **www.HealYourLife.com®** to regroup, recharge, and reconnect with your own magnificence.Featuring blogs, mind-body-spirit news, and life-changing wisdom from Louise Hay and friends.

Visit **www.HealYourLife.com** today!

HEAL YOUR LIFE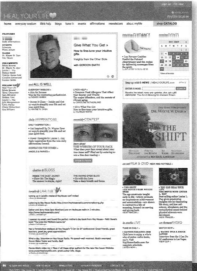

Take Your Soul on a Vacation

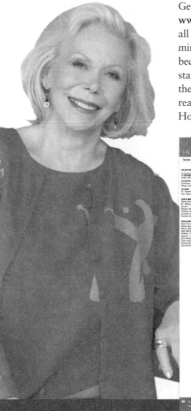

Get your daily dose of inspiration today at **www.HealYourLife.com®**. Brimming with all of the necessary elements to ease your mind and educate your soul, this Website will become the foundation from which you'll start each day. This essential site delivers the latest in mind, body, and spirit news and real-time content from your favorite Hay House authors.

Make It Your Home Page Today!

www.HealYourLife.com®